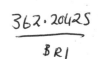

Acute Mental Health Care
in the Community
Intensive Home Treatment

Acute Mental Health Care in the Community

Intensive Home Treatment

Edited by

NEIL BRIMBLECOMBE BSc, MSc, RMN

West Hertfordshire Community NHS Trust

W

WHURR PUBLISHERS

LONDON AND PHILADELPHIA

© 2001 Whurr Publishers Ltd
First published 2001
by Whurr Publishers Ltd
19b Compton Terrace
London N1 2UN England and
325 Chestnut Street, Philadelphia PA 19106 USA

British Library Cataloguing in Publication Data

A catalogue record for this book
is available from the British Library.

ISBN 1 86156 189 X

Printed and bound in the UK by Athenaeum Press Ltd,
Gateshead, Tyne & Wear.

Contents

Preface

Studies investigating the viability of intensive home treatment as an alternative to admission have been appearing in the professional literature for over thirty years. There is now little disagreement that such services are feasible. They can provide, at the very least, care as effective as inpatient-focused services to a majority of individuals with severe, acute mental health problems. From a few pioneering examples, often set up as research projects, services have multiplied across the country although in a notably haphazard fashion. It is therefore timely that a volume should appear which explores in more detail the day-to-day issues inherent in providing such a service as a routine part of comprehensive mental health care provision.

This book aims to clarify the history of the development of these services and attempts to look for common themes amongst the myriad of structures that exist, to look at some clinical approaches adopted and then to explore a range of contextual factors affecting the setting up and day-to-day running of such services.

This book is written for all those providing or planning to provide intensive home treatment services, for those numerous mental health professionals who will come into contact with such services on a daily basis and for those studying for the mental health professions.

Neil Brimblecombe

Contributors

Patrick J Bracken, MA, MD, MRCPsych, DPM, PhD, is a Senior Research Fellow (University of Bradford) and Consultant Psychiatrist currently working to develop practical alternatives to institutional psychiatry for an inner-city population in Bradford. He has an interest in conceptual aspects of Psychiatry and holds doctorates in both Psychiatry and Philosophy. He has published widely on the topic of trauma and is co-editor, with Celia Petty, of the book *Rethinking the Trauma of War* (London: Free Association Books, 1998). With his colleague Phil Thomas, he writes a regular column called Postpsychiatry in the journal Open Mind.

Neil Brimblecombe, BSc, MSc, RMN, Dip NEBSMS, is Nurse Advisor/Clinical Governance Co-ordinator for the West Herts Community NHS Trust. He had previously managed and developed home treatment teams in the area for seven years, publishing several articles on the work of these services. He is currently completing doctoral studies into the effect of home treatment services on service outcomes.

Bruce Cohen, BSc(Hons), MSc, PhD, is a Marie Curie Research Fellow at the Humboldt Universität in Berlin. As well as work within the mental health arena he has also researched issues of crime, social housing, drug-taking, and safety in cities. His doctoral thesis on mental health user narratives led to a number of published articles.

Louise Dunn, MSc, CQSW, is a Senior Practitioner and approved social worker in a Community Mental Health team in Hertfordshire. Her present job involves working with clients with severe and enduring mental health problems, and promoting awareness of research which effects front-line practice. She has worked for social services in both generic and mental health teams, and been an approved social worker since 1991. She obtained a MSc in Mental Health Social Work at the Institute of Psychiatry, her research thesis being on the effect of home treatment services on Mental Health Act admissions.

Sarah Orme, BSc(Hons) is a Research Fellow in the Psychology Division of the University of Wolverhampton. Her research interests include the provision and organisation of crisis services and the evaluation of mental health services in general. She has previously published on the effectiveness of crisis services. Current projects include looking at multidisciplinary working in crisis teams, the effect of integrated care pathways in inpatient acute mental health care and developing a number of projects with local NHS and Social Services colleagues.

Introduction

NEIL BRIMBLECOMBE

After several decades of a stated policy of shifting the focus of care for those with mental health problems from the psychiatric hospital to the community, the situation in the UK remains one of widely varying services, and, indeed, attitudes. The rate at which community care has been developed has been slower than expected due to a range of issues, from inadequate funding to professional inertia to hostility from the media.

Sadly the phrase 'community care isn't working' seems to be widely accepted as a truism (Rose 1997, DoH 1998), although through frequency of repetition as much as serious analysis. It is doubtless true that the comprehensiveness and quality of mental health care provision does still vary widely from area to area. However, this also ignores the improved circumstances of many people with severe mental health problems, who in years gone by would have received either negligible care in their homes or long and isolating stays in an institution due to a lack of realistic alternatives.

This book will focus on a key aspect of comprehensive community-focused mental health care, that of intensive home treatment as an alternative to psychiatric admission for people with acute and severe mental health problems. The phrase intensive home treatment (IHT) is here taken to refer to any service:

- open for longer than normal office hours
- providing rapid assessment to individuals potentially requiring admission to acute psychiatric facilities
- offering home treatment where possible (normally in the form of relatively frequent home visits) as an alternative to hospitalisation.

1

Such services may utilise hospital admission at points during care, but their focus is on treatment in the community.

Many of the early projects in IHT were relatively short lived affairs, set up primarily as research projects, often with especially highly motivated and energetic staff. This book attempts to focus on the services subsequent to, and based on aspects of, the experience of those early pioneers. These services are those provided by 'ordinary' staff in 'ordinary' areas.

The stance of this editor is one of enthusiasm for the general principles of 'community care', but I am anxious to ensure that such care is as safe, effective and efficient as is possible. This is not a book which ignores the problems inherent in providing acute care in the community. For example, important questions have been raised concerning the safety of clients (Morgan 1992), the diversion of services from their original aims (Kwakwa 1995) and evidence that simply seeing clients more often does not necessarily improve outcomes (Muijen et al 1994).

This book also does not decry the use of admission to psychiatric wards per se, but rather supports the concept that care should be provided in the least restrictive environment possible to meet the health care needs of the client and to allow the management of risk to both client and others.

Besides IHT, other approaches to providing acute community care clearly have an important part to play in providing realistic alternatives to admission. For example, day hospitals (e.g. Creed 1995) and various forms of residential service (Stroul 1988) and crisis accommodation (Turkington, Kingdon and Malcolm 1991), either on their own, or in addition to IHT services, are important resources for those with severe, acute mental health problems. They are, however, outside of the remit of this book.

The first chapter provides a brief history of the development of community care in general and IHT services in particular. In Chapter 2 Sarah Orme provides a valuable description of the current numbers, structures and aims of home treatment services. In Chapter 3 the large amount of research in the home treatment field is discussed and critiqued by Bruce Cohen and Sarah Orme.

In relation to the actual delivery of home treatment in the community, Chapter 4 describes the process of assessment in an acute community setting. Chapter 5 is a research-based discussion, by Louise Dunn, on the role of home treatment teams in relation to the Mental Health Act. The following chapter considers the feasibility of working with individuals with suicidal ideation in a community setting, before going on to suggest a range of interventions.

The remaining chapters cover the setting up and development of home treatment services. In Chapter 7 Pat Bracken raises the importance of the philosophy of home treatment teams and then goes on to describe a team who have attempted to work, to a degree, with a conceptual framework different from that of much of contemporary psychiatry. Bruce Cohen then provides an insight into how this same team managed to develop despite a range of internal and inter-agency challenges. This case study illustrates the range of issues likely to be encountered in setting up any new team, whether radical in outlook or not. The final chapter attempts to resummarise the evidence for the continued expansion of IHT teams and then goes on to discuss the range of issues and problems which need to be addressed in order for any service to survive and flourish.

Although the structure of this book follows a logical progression, with chapters planned to build on the previous ones, each chapter has also been written in a manner which will allow it to be read alone, inevitably leading to a limited amount of repetition of key information.

References

Creed F (1995) Acute day hospital care. In: Phelan M, Strathdee G, Thornicroft G (eds) Emergency Mental Health Services in the Community. Cambridge: Cambridge University Press.

Department of Health (1998) Modernising Mental Health. Safe, sound and supportive. London: Department of Health.

Kwakwa J (1995) Alternatives to hospital-based mental health care. Nursing Times 91(23):38–39.

Morgan G (1992) Suicide prevention. Hazards on the fast lane to community care. British Journal of Psychiatry 160:149–153.

Muijen M, Cooney M, Strathdee G, Bell R, Hudson A (1994) Community psychiatric nurse teams: intensive support versus generic care. British Journal of Psychiatry 165:211–217.

Rose D (1997) Trial by television. Community Care 4–10 December 30–31.

Stroul BA (1988) Residential crisis services: a review. Hospital and Community Psychiatry 39(10):1095–1099.

Turkington D, Kingdon D, Malcolm K (1991) The use of an unstaffed flat for crisis intervention and rehabilitation. Psychiatric Bulletin 15:13–14.

CHAPTER 1

Community care and the development of intensive home treatment services

NEIL BRIMBLECOMBE

Summary

The move away from asylum-based care for the mentally ill and the reasons for this development are described. The origins of IHT services are described and research in this and related fields summarised. The question of how far community care has progressed is discussed.

The past few years have seen a marked growth in mental health services providing extended hours services with an explicit or implicit aim of reducing acute admissions to psychiatric wards (see Orme, Chapter 2, this volume). Such developments can rightly be seen as part of the general transfer in resources from inpatient to community-based care, although there is marked variation in level of provision from area to area and the focus and organisation of such services.

Mental health services are 'shaped by what has gone on before' (Thomas 1998). The structure, approach and beliefs of particular services are inevitably affected by the events and ideas which have contributed to their creation. This chapter briefly describes some of the historical features which have ultimately allowed the development of modern services that provide intensive home-based care for those with severe, acute mental health problems, and reviews selected relevant research.

The growth of asylums

In the second half of the nineteenth century there was a marked increase in the numbers of mental hospitals or asylums in England, France and the US. Until relatively recently this system has continued to provide most psychiatric care. A wide range of factors have been identified as leading to this development, including industrialisation, urbanisation, the increased complexity of community organisation, the weakening of traditional family and local community ties, rural–urban migration and the factory system geared to production (Pasamanick et al 1967). Additional to these social factors was the growth of the belief that treating the mentally ill in an asylum away from the rest of society could be positively therapeutic (Shorter 1997). Related to this idea was the rise of the psychiatric profession itself, whose growth and influence was initially tied to the well-being of the asylum system (Porter 1990).

Reid (1989) relates the establishment of asylums to the growth of a national market economy and a more centralised state. With the increase in wage labour and working outside of the home, the traditional pattern of 'coping and containment strategies' within the family were undermined and the state began to take on a greater role in policing and controlling people's behaviour. As the poor law relief system was both 'ideologically incompatible' with the need for the supply of cheap labour and was becoming too expensive for parishes to maintain, the 1834 Poor Law Amendment Act centralised the system. The 'mad' interfered with the smooth running of the workhouses, so an alternative needed to be found. The County Asylums Act of 1808 allowed for public asylums to be paid for and built. The 1845 Lunacy Acts made this compulsory.

Despite the efforts of various reformers, such as Tuke in England, Rush in the US and Pinel in France, standards of care and treatment remained generally low. Improvements in physical care ensured that hospital populations were not reduced markedly by infectious disease. However, there was no corresponding improvement in the treatment of the mental illnesses of those admitted, until the introduction of effective treatments for tertiary syphilis and the partial successes of electroconvulsive therapy (ECT).

The move away from asylums

Although the policy of the removal of the mentally ill to large asylums was questioned in various countries from the early years of this century, the mental hospital population continued to grow in most western countries until the 1940s and 1950s (Tyrer 1995). This radically changed from the 1950s onwards with many developed countries adopting policies, at least theoretically, dominated by variants of community care replacing hospital care and culminating in the closure of large hospitals (Kluiter 1997). The speed of this change was considered as nothing short of 'astonishing' by some (Pasamanick et al 1967).

In the UK, the 1930 Mental Treatment Act allowed for voluntary admission to psychiatric hospitals, with certain restrictions. It also allowed for the setting up of outpatient clinics, although, in reality, these were not widespread (Freeman 1999). In fact there had been a long history of isolated attempts at providing a degree of care in a community setting, e.g. a domiciliary crisis intervention service for mentally ill people at Barnhill Hospital in Glasgow in 1880 and an outpatient clinic at St Thomas's Hospital in London in 1889 although the first day hospital was not established until 1948 (Shorter 1997). Some schemes radically reorganised the focus of care away from large mental hospitals. In Manchester in 1948 psychiatrists were recruited who had a defined population to provide care for. This was provided through outpatient clinics and the use of beds in the three local general hospitals (Freeman 1999).

An early and striking experiment in community-focused care took place in 1956, when the South West Metropolitan Regional Hospital Board decided to instigate an outpatient and domiciliary treatment service in the coastal town of Worthing (Carse et al 1958). The reasons were the increasing number of admissions to overcrowded hospitals and concerns that they would soon be unable to meet the demands placed upon them. Also influential was the idea that hospital admission might lead the patient to 'run away from his problems' rather than resolve them.

The service provided consisted of an 'active treatment centre' and day hospital, staffed by psychiatric nurses and an occupational therapist. Outpatient clinics and home visits were provided by psychiatrists and two staff carried out social work. Treatments included

ECT, modified insulin therapy, brief psychotherapy and drug abre-action. Only deep insulin-shock treatment and prefrontal leucotomy were confined to hospital use. The number of admissions fell by 59% and 77% in the two hospitals which received admission from the area. The authors concluded that 'for a large proportion of psychiatric patients, admission is unnecessary and outpatient treatment can be entirely effective'.

These projects, however, were the exception rather than the rule. Care remained largely based on inpatient care in large asylums. Psychiatrists were generally poorly trained and psychiatric nurses underpaid and unappreciated (Freeman 1999). The first community psychiatric nursing posts, the professional group which remains the largest of those providing community-based care today, were not established until the 1950s (May and Moore 1963).

Following on from the findings of the Royal Commission on Mental Health Law, the Mental Health Act 1959, introduced the 'informal' admission, 'one of the historic events in psychiatric evolution in this country' (Macmillan 1963). This was seen as moving the 'centre of gravity' of psychiatric services towards the community (Macmillan 1963), and encouraged the treatment of patients in the community (Grad and Sainsbury 1968).

This Act, at the time, was in advance of public opinion and also of the views of many in the medical profession. A principal concern behind the 1959 act was to keep inpatient treatment to a minimum, and, as a consequence, to return the patient as soon as possible to the care of the community (Rollin 1977). However, there was no obligation placed on local authorities to provide community mental health services, nor was specific money forthcoming for this purpose (Freeman 1999).

The White Paper *Better Services for the Mentally Ill* (HMSO 1975) further emphasised the desirability of a shift from hospital-based to community-based services, an approach which has remained largely unchanged since (Tyrer 1995). However, the degree to which psychiatrists and other mental health care professions were also in agreement with this movement is doubtful. Cooper (1990) archly comments that 'nobody knows' who provided the detailed advice upon which *Better Services for the Mentally Ill* was based.

The White Paper prescribed what would constitute desirable components of a local mental health service, including a general hospital psychiatric unit for the treatment of acute episodes of mental distress, with at least five inpatient beds per 100 000 head of population. This unit should provide day and inpatient treatment and be a base from which 'specialist therapeutic teams provide advice and consultation outside the hospital'. There was also greater responsibility to be placed on social services for the provision of social care in the community: day care, social clubs and residential care. This shift was reinforced in the Mental Health Act (HMSO 1983) which described the duty 'for health and social services authorities . . . to provide after care'.

Reasons for the shift towards community-based care

The causes of the shift from hospital-based to community-based services are complicated and, to a large extent, unclear (Fenton et al 1982, Reid 1989), with different commentators citing different factors. These include:

- antipsychotic medication
- financial considerations
- professional gain
- change in 'psychiatric discourse'
- rejection of institutions
- growth in the 'user' movement.

Antipsychotic medication

The most commonly cited reason for the move towards more community-based care is the introduction of antipsychotic medication in 1953 and its almost universal use since 1955. It has been claimed that it led to less need for hospitalisation and 'probably had a more profound effect on the mental hospital as an institution and as part of a community care program than all the other changes combined' (Pasamanick et al 1967). However, others argue that the effect of antipsychotic medication may have been 'vastly overvalued' (Eisenberg 2000). Certainly it appears that early optimism about the efficacy of such drugs soon diminished (Jones 1972).

Rollin (1977) expresses doubts about the overall efficacy of psychotropic medications in so far as 'what they seem incapable of doing with any degree of certainty is to prevent relapses'. Certainly there had been some success in markedly reducing admissions by community intervention prior to the availability of antipsychotics. A notable example was the situation in Amsterdam in the 1930s as described by Querido (1968). A 'psychiatric first aid service' was developed which provided a 24-hour on-the-spot assessment of anyone for whom hospital admission was requested. Querido estimated that about 10% of the 1930s Amsterdam hospital population and 50% of 'first aid' patients could live in the community provided certain conditions were met. These included 'medical treatment and expert supervision' but (especially for the hospital residents) were chiefly of a 'simple, material nature: a home, a bed, clothes'.

Scull (1977) also points out that the general policy of de-institutionalisation was applied to groups where the efficacy of antipsychotic medication was largely irrelevant, such as the elderly and the mentally handicapped.

Financial considerations

Various commentators (e.g. Reid 1989) have suggested that the cost of maintaining the asylum system was a significant factor in its demise. Scull (1977) strongly argues that the move to community care can be seen largely in fiscal terms, with governments since the Second World War having needed to curb ever-increasing welfare spending. However, Busfield (1986) claims that such an argument is not supported by policies in the 1950s and 1960s, but arguably does in terms of the attempts at cost cutting by successive governments in the 1970s and 1980s.

Prior (1991) concludes that the economic argument for a switch to community care is flawed. There is no evidence that initial planners of the move (for example, in *Better Services for the Mentally Ill* 1975) consciously considered such a move to be cost cutting. Nor is there evidence that cost cutting has been consistently achieved since that time. However, whether it is a valid argument or not, in attempting to justify the more radical moves towards community care, such as with IHT as an alternative to admission, proponents have tended to be careful to justify this on grounds of financial efficiency as well as clinical and client satisfaction (Langsley et al 1968, Weisbrod, Test and Stein 1980, Punukollu 1991, Burns et al 1993, Knapp et al 1994, Minghella et al 1998).

Professional gain

Several authors (e.g. Mosher 1983, Kennedy 2000) have commented on the benefit to psychiatrists of moving from the asylums into inpatient units based in general hospitals. In this way psychiatry has been conceptualised as seeking a 'rapprochement' with the rest of medicine. Pasamanick et al (1967) described the situation in the US where psychiatrists had an investment in the transfer of care from the stigmatised state hospitals to the community, in terms both of opportunities for financial remuneration and of improving the low standing of psychiatry compared with other medical specialities.

Although such an argument would, to a degree, explain the shift from large asylums to units in district general hospitals, it would not support a further move to more community-focused care. In fact, such a rationale might explain some reluctance to shift away from such smaller institutions, which would lead to a further separation of psychiatry from the more prestigious hospital-based medical specialities, a 'disruption of its new relation with the rest of medicine' (Mosher 1983).

Change in 'psychiatric discourse'

Prior (1991) sees the most satisfactory explanation for the shift away from institutional care to be related to a change in psychiatric discourse. He describes the manner in which the incorporation of psychological means of understanding, both behavioural and psychodynamic, into psychiatric training and practice simply no longer fitted with care provided in large institutions. The treatment of large numbers of soldiers with 'shell shock' in the First World War had introduced psychodynamic ideas to psychiatrists. 'Social psychiatry', with its examination of the non-somatic factors and social relationships involved in acute illness, clearly existed most easily in a community setting. This became linked with the idea that one cannot cure a mentally ill individual at the same time that he or she is segregated from society (Eaton 1986).

However, although some psychiatrists played important roles in propounding that care could, and indeed should, be given in non-institutional settings (Freeman 1999), this was often far from the case, with Reid (1989) portraying psychiatrists as having a vested interest in maintaining services in hospital settings. Murphy (1992) states that 'psychiatrists have not on the whole played the role originally expected of them in the closure of hospitals and the development of community alternatives', and Simpson (1993) describes the traditional view of hospital consultants that quantity of beds is a 'reflection of their own machismo'.

Although Prior emphasises the 'demedicalisation of psychiatry' as being of significance, his argument ignores the recent resurgent focus in psychiatry on biological interventions and the disturbing prospect of social and psychological aspects of care being increasingly disregarded (Clare 1999). Even apparently non-medical interventions, such as working with families of those with schizophrenia, can be characterised as reinforcing a medical model of psychiatric illness (e.g. Johnstone 1993). However, these reservations do not dismiss Prior's central argument that 'modern psychiatry' no longer requires an emphasis on inpatient care, as tablets can be taken anywhere.

Rejection of institutions

A series of descriptive publications portrayed a bleak and damaging life inside mental institutions (Barton 1959, Goffman 1968). Mental hospitals were seen as being, by their very nature, harmful, and therefore living outside the hospital, with the aid of psychotropic drugs, would be 'inherently more therapeutic' (Fenton et al 1982). After the Second World War any total institution inevitably had connotations of the concentration camp, 'the symbol of ultimate evil' (Pasamanick et al 1967). Furthermore, due to the rise of the welfare state there was no longer any need for individuals to enter institutions just in order to receive care, food and shelter, as had been the case in the previous century.

Generally, the gradual acceptance in society of some psychoanalytic ways of understanding mental illness increased acceptance of the mentally ill on the grounds that they were only somewhat more damaged than the rest of neurotic humanity. So by the mid-1950s a prominent US psychiatrist could claim that: 'Gone forever is the notion that the mentally ill person is the exception. It is now accepted that most people have some degree of mental illness at some time, and many of them have a degree of mental illness most of the time' (Menninger 1963). Meanwhile, equal rights movements pressed forward the concept of a single humanity, the arguments for which could be broadly applied across all groups in society.

Pasamanick et al comment about the speed of the switch from hospital-focused to community-focused services, but point out that

> this movement is a tribute not nearly as much to faith in community programs per se as to a revolt against the mental hospital as a treatment center. The mental hospital may perhaps never again have the leading mental health role it once held (1967, p. 6).

Cooper (1990) contends that the decisions taken to move the focus of care from hospital to community were not arrived at by means of evaluative studies, nor by examination of the needs of the community or even by considering the views of the psychiatrists, rather they were adopted because 'they seemed reasonable and attractive from several points of view, and because they have a very obviously humane feel about them'.

Growth in the 'user' movement

Peck and Jenkins (1992) cite the growth of the mental health service user movement as likely to contribute significantly in the future to the development of community-based approaches, such as crisis intervention, community treatment and assertive outreach. They see the growth of this movement as the result of two different social trends. The first emphasises the importance of 'oppressed individuals' meeting to discuss the causes and the effects of the oppression that they are experiencing. This is seen as being traceable back to the 'consciousness-raising' approaches of civil rights groups in the US. The second trend again originates from the US, this time from the work of Ralph Nader which stressed the importance of the consumer in a free-market economy. A third influence which could be added is that of the 'anti-psychiatry' movement, characterised by the diverse views of such as Laing (e.g. 1960) and Szasz (e.g. 1972). Nasser (1995) portraying the user movement as being, at least partially, an 'offshoot' of anti-psychiatry.

In relation to the potential influence users of services may now have, 'consumerism' within the NHS has certainly given an opportunity for increasing user representation in the decision-making process at health board and trust levels (Cohen 1998). Structural changes in the commissioning of mental health services may also have contributed to giving users more of a voice in the focus of services. Part of the purchasing role of health agencies as ascertaining local health needs can involve consultation with GPs, carers and the users themselves.

There is, however, no evidence that service users were directly influential in the development of early policies moving towards more community-based care. This situation has since changed with greater publicity given to users' views (although rarely as much as that given to relatives). The wishes of users have been cited in the development of a number of community-focused and crisis services. User satisfaction surveys have consistently been used to help justify the continued existence of community services (e.g. Marks et al 1994, Coleman et al 1998, Minghella et al 1998, Cohen 1999).

The interplay of all the above factors contributed, in varying degrees, to a situation where there was at least the possibility of beginning to establish community-based services, instead of the former reliance on asylum-based care. Pioneering services, focusing on non-hospital-based interventions, then began to set precedents, backed up by research which led towards the establishment of today's acute IHT teams.

Home treatment services

In attempting to explore the roots of current home treatment services three broad influences can be identified:

- Firstly, the general move towards community care in the UK, including some of the ground-breaking services described above.
- Secondly, services espousing variants of a crisis intervention philosophy, commonly providing brief interventions to prevent admission or intervene in 'psychiatric emergencies'.
- Thirdly, services concerned at the negative effects of hospital admission, which also aimed at reducing 'secondary impairment' in the community by providing home treatment, and, often, extended follow-up, as an alternative to admission.

In reality the division between the last two categories has often been blurred, as described below.

Crisis theory and crisis intervention teams

The 'crisis intervention' philosophy of care has been highly influential in its various practical interpretations. This has occasionally been incorporated into the rationale for IHT services, although was often absent from the writings of some of the pioneers of home treatment services in the UK (Dean and Gadd 1990, Muijen et al 1992).

Crisis theory developed largely from the work of Lindemann (1944) who studied the reactions of the survivors of a fire disaster at the Coconut Grove Nightclub in Boston. However, it was the work of Gerald Caplan which popularised crisis theory as a way of understanding mental and behavioural disturbance and how and when interventions could be made to help the individual. Caplan saw a crisis as occurring when an individual is faced with an obstacle to important life goals and customary problem-solving methods are ineffective at dealing with it (Caplan 1964). During the subsequent short period of disorganisation, the individual was particularly open to receiving help which potentially allows the individual to emerge from the crisis at a higher level of functioning than that at which they began.

The Denver study: crisis intervention in the US

There is a strong history of services in the US which share with others the essential aim of preventing unnecessary admission, but do so from a crisis intervention theoretical standpoint, utilising a family systems approach (e.g. Rubenstein 1972, Bengelsdorf and Alden 1987). The premise of these services is that signs of a psychiatric disorder in an individual may be accompanied by or reflect a breakdown or a disorder in a system of which the client is a part.

One of the most striking services utilising such an approach, and which inspired many later pioneers, was found in Denver from 1964 onwards (Langsley et al 1969). Three hundred patients seen as requiring admission to psychiatric facilities were randomly assigned to either outpatient 'family crisis therapy' (FCT) or were admitted. To qualify for the study patients had to live in a family within an hour's drive. The treatment provided focused on here-and-now problems, and relationships within the family. Medication was given to any family member apparently requiring it. Mean treatment period was 24.2 days.

The FCT group was found to be less likely to be hospitalised in a 6 month period after treatment, and periods of hospitalisation were shorter. They also scored well on scales of social adaptation and successful management of crises. The cost of FCT was estimated to be less than one-sixth that of hospital treatment. The authors concluded that FCT was an effective alternative to hospitalisation for individuals living in a family and traditionally seen as hospitalisable (Langsley et al 1971).

The most striking finding of all was that not one of the 150 cases in the FCT group required admission at any time during the treatment period, despite including 'acutely disturbed schizophrenics, suicidal depressive and other dramatic behavioral disturbances'. The authors were at pains, however, to point out that a small number of admission beds would always be needed, particularly for some of those already accustomed to using hospital as a way of solving problems and those not living with a family.

Crisis intervention in the UK

With the dramatic results reported from 'crisis' services such as that described by Langsley and his colleagues in Denver, it was not surprising that services following variants of a crisis intervention philosophy spread. In England a few areas established services which proved to be relatively long lived, with Barnet as a forerunner, to be followed by Coventry, Tower Hamlets, Lewisham and Tunbridge Wells. Most of these areas produced some research that helped to support their continuing existence. Both Coventry and Tower Hamlets utilised client satisfaction studies, finding high levels of satisfaction among clients and a preference for crisis intervention treatment rather than hospital admission (Davis et al 1985, Parkes 1992). However, what is less clear is whether these clients were those who would normally require admission, with one study showing that the majority of clients perceived their problems to be related to depression, sometimes with ideas of self-harm, loneliness and relationship problems (Davis et al 1985).

In Barnet, Lawrence Ratna's service offered a 24-hour urgent assessment service by a multidisciplinary team where there was 'urgent demand for immediate psychiatric intervention'. He was able to claim that for a client group aged over 65, fewer long-term admissions took place as a result of the availability of this service, in addition to other follow-up focusing on social aspects of care (Ratna 1982).

Problems with 'crisis intervention'

Caplan's stereotypical patient was one who was a previously well-adjusted individual. What became clear relatively early on was that such a patient as this was the exception rather than the rule in crisis services. Cooper (1979) found few such individuals being dealt with by crisis units he visited in a study of European crisis services:

> almost universal disappointment was found in the extent to which the patients coming forward fit the ideal or stereotypical patient implied in most crisis theories. The previously well adjusted person needing constructive help during a severe crisis is quite rare in ordinary civil practice.

This study suggested that the theoretical basis for crisis work might be seriously challenged in practice (Lee 1990). However, exponents of crisis theory and its variants have been keen to justify its use even with the most chronically disturbed individuals.

In 1985 Tufnell and his colleagues described the working of the Lewisham Crisis Intervention Team. Referrals were accepted for 'psychiatric emergencies', requiring urgent admission or urgent treatment beyond the referrer's resources. Although they only operated an assessment service during office hours they were able to offer daily visits following assessment. What is particularly striking is that the authors generally saw the notion of 'crisis intervention' as problematic, stating that they preferred to discuss their service in terms of 'home assessment and treatment'. A later review of the work of this service estimated that only 12% of referrals could be seen as 'classic crisis' type clients (Beer et al 1995).

Some services styled as 'crisis intervention teams' have little in common with their predecessors, for example the Aintree Crisis Management Team in Liverpool is only able to see those who are already known to mental health services and are on the higher levels of the care programme approach (CPA) (Crompton 1997). Even though arguments are made that a crisis intervention model is still of value in working with clients with enduring, severe mental health problems, such services undoubtedly do not attempt to provide the framework which early proponents believed would actually prevent such problems becoming established in the first place.

The Madison study

Although some services focused on the benefits of applying crisis theory, others were more concerned with the potential damage caused by hospital admission and the need to prevent 'secondary impairments' in the community. Of these services undoubtedly the most influential have been those set up in Dane County, Madison, Wisconsin by Leonard Stein and colleagues (Stein, Test and Marx 1975, Stein and Test 1980, Weisbrod, Test and Stein 1980, Test and Stein 1980). They utilised a randomised control methodology to divide patients presenting for admission at the local psychiatric hospital into one of two groups. The first were normally admitted and received hospital-based treatment with outpatient follow-up. The second were rarely admitted and received home treatment in the form of 'training for community living' (TCL) for a 14-month period.

Under this programme staff were available 24 hours a day. There was an emphasis on assistance with daily living activities, such as cooking and personal hygiene. Sheltered workshops were provided for employment. General 'support' was given to the patient and carers. Medication was routinely used for patients diagnosed as schizophrenic or manic-depressive. A range of clinical and social functioning rating scales were used at the initial assessment and periodically through the following months of treatment. The study found that after 12 months the TCL treatment group, as compared with the control group, had spent significantly less time in hospital and less time unemployed, had more contact with 'trusted friends', were more satisfied with their life situations and had less symptomatology overall. The control group did not do significantly better than the TCL group on any scale.

Although this and other similar studies (Fenton et al 1982, Hoult et al 1984) achieved impressive results and were able to conclude that psychiatric care for those with severe, acute mental health problems did not necessarily mean hospital care, they had not been carried out in the UK. There had therefore been no chance to formally attempt such an approach in the British social, cultural and medical climate. A pioneering although relatively small scale home treatment service had been set up in Birmingham and had been successful at reducing admission rates and hospital lengths of stay (Dean and Gadd 1990) through adopting some of the techniques from Madison, and the limited amount of research from crisis intervention teams suggested positive results for services offering a degree of alternative to admission.

The Southwark study

Inspired by the example of such programmes as that in Madison, the creators of the Daily Living Programme in Southwark set up an ambitious study (Muijen et al 1992, Marks et al 1994). Individuals referred for emergency admission in the Southwark area of London were randomly selected for either home-based care by the Daily Living Programme (DLP) team, consisting predominantly of community psychiatric nurses and psychiatrists, or standard inpatient treatment (followed up by outpatients). Although most of the home treatment group were admitted at some point during the 20-month follow-up period, overall the number of inpatient bed days was greatly less than in the control group. This advantage was later lost when the home treatment team lost control over discharges from the wards.

Various measures were made after 4, 11 and 20 months, although it is notable that many of the home treatment group were still inpatients at the 4-month stage. Clinical improvement in the two groups were similar, with the home treatment patients scoring significantly better after 20 months. Patient and relative satisfaction was higher in the home treatment group, although only significant after 11 months.

The trial was not without incident; several suicides and a murder took place in the home treatment group. Although it later appeared that high suicide rates were to be found across the whole local area, it was also clear that providing home treatment as an alternative to admission was a difficult and risky endeavour, although not necessarily more so than providing mental health care in traditional fashion (Connolly et al 1996). What was different about community-based services seemed to be that they were more vulnerable to trial by media if something went wrong.

Current home treatment services

Of all the projects described above, those of Stein and his colleagues in Madison have probably been the most influential for those interested in developing community-focused mental health services. However, planners have chosen to focus on differing aspects of their work. Some have taken on those aspects relating to acute interventions with individuals as a short-term alternative to hospitalisation, but others have focused on different features. Thus today there is a related, but largely separate, approach focusing on 'Assertive Community Treatment' with an emphasis on working over extended periods of time with the long-term severely mentally ill using an 'assertive' approach, often with those who are rejecting of services (e.g. Craig and Pathare 1997). Treatment is potentially relatively intensive, with low client to staff ratios, but the focus is on longer-term engagement, rather than just the reduction of acute symptoms.

Acute, short-term home treatment services are currently found, for example, in Bradford, Manchester, North Birmingham and Hertfordshire. Although not utilising a crisis intervention framework with their clients, they do have certain similarities with crisis intervention teams, in that they aim to provide rapid early assessment and then give intensive short-term care only. They do not provide the longer-term follow-up exemplified in Madison and Southwark. Other services are expected to fulfil this role.

The acute home treatment team seems to have arisen for a number of different reasons. Individuals, most frequently consultant psychiatrists with a conviction that non-institutional care is the best option whenever possible, have been able to set up services largely through their own enthusiasm, with the ability to quote earlier studies to support these moves. In some areas this has been facilitated by pressure from service users to provide more alternatives to admission (Bailey 1994/95). O'Grady (1996) sees the issue of whether home treatment services are adopted locally as being down to the 'interplay of local voices' and 'the interplay between policy and its local interpretation, key voices in shaping services and the readiness of providers to alter existing service patterns'.

A common feature which has supported the development of home treatment services has been extreme pressure on inpatient beds. This has provided a context where the idea of providing alternatives to admission is appealing to local healthcare organisations. The reasons why acute home treatment seems to be favoured over a type which provides both acute and longer-term care are harder to discover, but most probably relate to the advantages of developing high levels of experience and skills in working with acute problems in a single team and not having to balance the resources of a large individual team between the need for continuing and acute care.

Research into acute IHT services

With such services still in their infancy, there is, as yet, relatively little research concerning IHT. What there is can be divided into those which compare client outcomes for those receiving home treatment as compared with those receiving other services such as hospital admission, and smaller-scale local studies describing services and analysing their effects.

Comparing outcomes between services

A study comparing outcomes between a service offering IHT and one that did not was carried out by the Sainsbury Centre in North Birmingham (Minghella et al 1998). The study examined the work of the Psychiatric Emergency Team (PET), which provided short-term 24-hour home care as an alternative to inpatient admission.

In a 45-week period outcomes and characteristics were compared for 200 clients in two Birmingham wards. The first ward provided 90 cases from admissions to hospital to the study, and the second provided 110 cases, consisting of one in three admissions to either an acute bed or referrals to the Psychiatric Emergency Team. There were no differences in symptomatic outcomes between the two groups, although a low response rate (35%) restricts the generalisability of this finding. The clients in the PET area had only 38.2% of the bed days of those in the comparison area. There were no major differences in the frequency of untoward events nor in rereferral rates to acute care. Most users were satisfied with the service they received and there was no significant difference between levels of satisfaction in the two areas. The cost of care in the PET area was found to be significantly cheaper, although this only included the costs of mental health services, excluding the costs to other agencies.

Other acute IHT research

A frequent focus has been on user satisfaction with studies finding high levels of satisfaction with home treatment services and, where asked, the majority of clients preferring home treatment to hospital admission (Kwakwa 1995, Godfrey 1996, Coleman et al 1998, Cohen 1999).

The effect on admission rates of the introduction of home treatment services has been evaluated in a number of areas (Whittle and Mitchell 1997) with significant reductions usually found. However, exceptions have been noted when a service has begun to focus on those client groups not normally admitted to hospital (Kwakwa 1995).

In areas with home treatment teams, comparisons have been made between characteristics of clients treated at home and those admitted to hospital. Individuals admitted to the wards have been found to be more likely to present with 'attention-seeking behaviour', bizarre speech content, overactivity or socially unacceptable behaviour (Harrison et al 1999). In some areas higher than expected rates of admission have been found for individuals diagnosed with personality disorder (Bracken and Cohen 1999, Brimblecombe and O'Sullivan 1999), although the majority of all diagnostic categories appear to be treatable at home as opposed to hospital. The majority of clients with suicidal ideation also appear to be treatable at home (Harrison et al 1999, Brimblecombe 2000).

How far has community care progressed?

Having examined the reasons behind the shift of focus from institutional to community-based care, and the influences on the development of home treatment teams, it is important to provide an overview of how far this process has actually gone.

The number of NHS mental illness beds has reduced dramatically, from a peak of around 150 000 in the mid-1950s to a level of 38 780 by 1996–97 (DoH 1998a), although some of this reduction can be explained by transfer of long-stay beds to residential and private nursing homes. Despite these dramatic changes in numbers, more recently there appears to have been little shift in resources, with a similar proportion of around two-thirds being spent on inpatient care in 1997–98 (Health Select Committee 1998) as in 1992–93 (Audit Commission 1994).

Despite the White Papers, change following the recommendations was slow (Peck and Jenkins 1992), although some pioneering services were developed, for example the crisis intervention teams in Barnet and Coventry mentioned above. However, from the beginning of the 1980s there was a marked expansion in multidisciplinary teams with a community base (the community mental health centres). Throughout the decade their numbers doubled every two years, although their activities and facilities varied considerably (Sayce et al 1991), and they were usually only open during office hours and did not provide a comprehensive crisis service.

In terms of alternatives to psychiatric ward admission, by 1994 a survey carried out by the Sainsbury Centre for Mental Health (Faulkner et al 1994) indicated that only three (6.5%) of the 49 Health Authorities surveyed had mental health services providing such a service. A further three had residential alternatives to admission. However, at that point 11% of authorities were in the process of reviewing or discussing the development of a crisis service of some kind. Since that time new services have been set up in a number of areas or existing community services have increased their hours of operation in order to provide an out-of-hours service, although often limited to known service users. McMillan (1997) describes a 'dramatic rise' in many different forms of crisis services over the past few years, although considers the numbers available too few to adequately meet the potential need. Orme's study of crisis, home treatment and emergency services (see Chapter 2) confirms that this increase includes that of acute home treatment services offering alternatives to hospital admission.

After a long history of a conspicuous lack in clear 'top down' guidance from central government concerning the nature of services which should be provided in mental health (Rogers and Pilgrim 1996), there has been a recent flurry of activity in the DoH. The governmental stance expressed in *Modernising Mental Health. Safe, Sound and Supportive* (DoH 1998b), displayed a curious ambivalence towards community services, on the one hand arguing for increases in beds and proclaiming that community care has 'failed', yet on the other talking of the need for more crisis services, giving the North Birmingham service as an example of good practice. The National Service Framework for Mental Health (DoH 1999) seems generally more positive in tone, particularly in its encouragement for emergency services (although vague about their constitution). The

National Plan is more specific, with the exception of 335 'crisis resolution services' which should be created before 2004 (DoH 2000).

Conclusions: reinstitutionalisation or empowerment?

Even where moves have been made from the old asylums, there is a view that these changes were, at least at times, not so much deinstitutionalisation as reinstitutionalisation (Rogers and Pilgrim 1996). Large institutions have shut down, but these may have been replaced with smaller institutions: 'the medical hegemony continues . . . . Same philosophy, same ideology on various smaller sites . . . . Does this reflect the spirit of community care?' (Reid 1989). Even where community-based alternatives are established, in terms of home treatment as an alternative to admission, there may be a risk that they simply 'bring the institution into the community' (Bracken and Thomas 1999). The traditional psychiatric role of surveillance which previously largely existed only in hospital settings can be seen as becoming even more intrusive as it enters even into people's homes.

It is striking how rarely the pioneers of home treatment in this country have explicitly adopted an ideological stance in their publications. Whether this was as a deliberate position to reduce the likelihood of rejection by mainstream psychiatry, or simply that such an ideology was not present, is an interesting question. However, some proponents of home treatment clearly do have a specific agenda in trying to shift the ideological balance of mental health care away from institutional models and custodialism (Sashidharan 1994, Bracken and Thomas 1999, and Bracken, Chapter 7, this volume).

Home treatment in its current form is a recent development and is likely to continue to evolve over the next few years, responding to local needs, research findings and moves from central government. It offers much to many, particularly in terms of avoiding the stresses of inpatient care, allowing clients and their carers to maintain as much independence and privacy as possible and ensuring that inpatient resources are left available for those most in need of high levels of supervision. For staff, the non-institutional setting of home treatment provides an opportunity for creativeness in working practices, but also demands a willingness to negotiate from a position where the client has authority in their own home, as opposed to having little or none as in the traditional hospital setting.

References

Audini B, Marks I, Lawrence R, Connolly J, Watts V (1994) Home based versus out-patient/inpatient care for people with serious mental illness. Phase II of a controlled study. British Journal of Psychiatry 165:195–203.

Audit Commission (1994) Finding a Place. London: Audit Commission.

Bailey S (1994/95) Bradford crisis services. Where are they? Open Mind 72:15.

Barton WR (1959) Institutional Neurosis. Bristol: Wright.

Beer D, Cope S, Smith J, Smith R (1995) The crisis team as part of comprehensive local services. Psychiatric Bulletin 19:616–619.

Bengelsdorf H, Alden DC (1987) A mobile crisis unit in the psychiatric emergency room. Hospital and Community Psychiatry 38:662–665.

Bracken P, Cohen B (1999) Home treatment in Bradford. Psychiatric Bulletin 23:349–352.

Bracken P, Thomas P (1999) Home treatment in Bradford. Open Mind 95:17.

Brimblecombe N (2000) Suicidal ideation, home treatment and admission. Mental Health Nursing 20(1):22–26.

Brimblecombe N, O'Sullivan G (1999) Diagnosis, assessments and admissions from a community treatment team. Psychiatric Bulletin 23:72–74.

Burns T, Raferty J, Beadsmore A, McGuigan S, Dickson M (1993) A controlled trial of home-based acute psychiatric services. II: Treatment patterns and costs. British Journal of Psychiatry 163:55–61.

Busfield J (1986) Managing Madness: changing ideas and practice. London: Unwin Hyman.

Caplan G (1964) Principles of Preventive Psychiatry. London: Tavistock.

Carse J, Panton NE, Watt A (1958) A district mental health service. The Worthing experiment. Lancet 4 January:39–41.

Clare AW (1999) Psychiatry's future: Psychological medicine or biological psychiatry? Journal of Mental Health 8(2):109–111.

Cohen BMZ (1999) Evaluation of the Bradford Home Treatment Service: Final Report. Bradford: University of Bradford.

Cohen M (1998) Users' movement and the challenge to psychiatrists. Psychiatric Bulletin 22:155–157.

Coleman M, Donnelly P, Davies A, Brace P (1998) Evaluating intensive support in community mental health care. Mental Health Nursing 18(5):8–11.

Connolly J, Marks I, Lawrence R, McNamee G, Muijen M (1996) Observations from community care for serious mental illness during a controlled study. Psychiatric Bulletin 20:3–7.

Cooper JE (1979) Crisis admission units and emergency psychiatric services. Public Health in Europe, Vol 11. Copenhagen: World Health Organization.

Cooper JE (1990) Professional obstacles to implementation and diffusion of innovative approaches to mental health care. In: Marks IM, Scott RA (eds) Mental Health Care Delivery: innovations, impediments and implementation. Cambridge: Cambridge University Press.

Craig T, Pathare S (1997) Assertive community treatment for the severely mentally ill in West Lambeth. Advances in Psychiatric Treatment 3:111–118.

Crompton N (1997) Early intervention begins at home. Nursing Times 93(52):27–28.

Davis A, Newton S, Smith D (1985) Coventry Crisis Intervention Team: the consumer's view. Social Services Research 2(1):7–32.

Dean C, Gadd EM (1990) Home treatment for acute psychiatric illness. British Medical Journal 301:1021–1023.

DoH (1998a) Health and Personal Social Services Statistics for England 1997. London: Stationery Office.

DoH (1998b) Modernising Mental Health. Safe, Sound and Supportive. London: Department of Health.

DoH (1999) National Service Framework for Mental Health. Modern Standards and Service Models. London: Department of Health.

DoH (2000) The NHS Plan. London: Department of Health.

Eaton WW (1986) The Sociology of Mental Disorders, 2nd edn. New York: Praeger.

Eisenberg L (2000) Is psychiatry more mindful or brainier than it was a decade ago? British Journal of Psychiatry 176:1–5.

Faulkner A, Field V, Muijen M (1994) A Survey of Adult Mental Health Services. London: Sainsbury Centre.

Fenton F, Tessier L, Struening E, Smith F, Benoit C (1982) Home and Hospital Psychiatric Treatment. London: Croom Helm.

Freeman H (1999) Psychiatry in the National Health Service 1948–1998. British Journal of Psychiatry 175:3–11.

Godfrey M (1996) User and carer outcomes in mental health. Outcome briefings. Nuffield Institute for Health 8:17–20.

Goffman I (1968) Asylums. Harmondsworth: Pelican Books.

Grad J, Sainsbury P (1968) The effects that patients have on their families in a community care and a control psychiatric service – a two year follow-up. British Journal of Psychiatry 114:265–278.

Harrison J, Poynton A, Marshall J, Gater R, Creed F (1999) Open all hours: extending the role of the psychiatric day hospital. Psychiatric Bulletin 23:400–404.

Health Select Committee (1998) Public Expenditure Inquiry. London: HMSO.

HMSO (1975) Better Services for the Mentally Ill. Cmnd 6223. London: HMSO.

HMSO (1983) Mental Health Act 1983. London: HMSO.

Hoult J, Rosen A, Reynolds I (1984) Community orientated treatment compared to psychiatric hospital orientated treatment. Social Science and Medicine 18(11):1005–1010.

Johnstone L (1993) Family management in 'schizophrenia': its assumptions and contradictions. Journal of Mental Health 2:255–269.

Jones K (1972) A history of the mental health services. London: Routledge and Kegan Paul.

Kennedy P (2000) Is psychiatry losing touch with the rest of medicine? Advances in Psychiatric Treatment 6:16–21.

Kluiter H (1997) Inpatient treatment and care arrangements to replace or avoid it – searching for an evidence-based balance. Current Opinions in Psychiatry 10:160–167.

Knapp M, Beecham J, Koutsogeorgopoulou V et al (1994) Service use and costs of home-based versus hospital based care for people with serious mental illness. British Journal of Psychiatry 165:195–203.

Kwakwa J (1995) Alternatives to hospital-based mental health care. Nursing Times 91(23):38–39.

Laing RD (1960) The Divided Self: A Study of Sanity and Madness. London: Tavistock.

Langsley DG, Pittman FS, Machotka P, Flomenhaft K (1968) Family crisis therapy – results and implications. Family Process 7(2):145–158.

Langsley DG, Flomenhaft K, Machotka P (1969) Followup evaluation of family crisis therapy. American Journal of Orthopsychiatry 39(5):753–759.

Langsley DG, Machotka P, Flomenhaft K (1971) Avoiding mental hospital admission: a follow-up study. American Journal of Psychiatry 127(10):127–130.

Lee H (1990) Out-of-hours work by CPNs. In: Brooker C (ed) Community Psychiatric Nursing. A research perspective. London: Chapman and Hall.

Lindemann D (1944) Symptomatology and management of acute grief. American Journal of Psychiatry 101:141–148.

MacMillan D (1963) Recent developments in community mental health. Lancet 16 March:567–571.

Marks IM, Connolly J, Muijen M, Audini B, McNamee G, Lawrence RE (1994) Home-based versus hospital-based care for people with serious mental illness. British Journal of Psychiatry 165:179–194.

May AR, Moore S (1963) The mental nurse in the community. Lancet 26 January:213–214.

McMillan I (1997) Confidence in a crisis. Mental Health Practice 1:3.

Menninger K (1963) The Vital Balance: the life balance in mental health and illness. New York: Viking.

Minghella E, Ford R, Freeman T, Hoult J, McGlynn P, O'Halloran P (1998) Open All Hours. 24-hour response for people with mental health emergencies. London: Sainsbury Centre for Mental Health.

Mosher LR (1983) Alternatives to psychiatric hospitalization. Why has research failed to be translated into practice? New England Journal of Medicine 309(25):1579–1580.

Muijen M, Marks IM, Connolly J, McNamee G (1992) The Daily Living Programme. Preliminary comparison of community versus hospital-based treatment for the seriously mentally ill facing emergency admission. British Journal of Psychiatry 160:379–384.

Murphy E (1992) Resourcing for the future: the balance of revenue in community services. In: Peck E (ed) Community Mental Health Services: Models for the Future. Conference Proceedings No. 11, University of Newcastle upon Tyne Health Services Management Unit.

Nasser M (1995) The rise and fall of anti-psychiatry. Psychiatric Bulletin 19:743–746.

O'Grady JC (1996) Community psychiatry: central policy, local implementation. British Journal of Psychiatry 169:259–262.

Parkes CM (1992) Perceptions of a crisis service by referrers and clients. Psychiatric Bulletin 16:751–753.

Pasamanick B, Scarpitti FR, Dinitz S (1967) Schizophrenics in the Community: an experimental study in the prevention of hospitalization. New York: Appleton-Century-Crofts.

Peck E, Jenkins J (1992) The development of acute psychiatric crisis services in England: Opportunities, problems and trends. Journal of Mental Health 1:193–200.

Porter R (1990) Mind-Forg'd Manacles. Harmondsworth: Penguin Books.

Prior L (1991) Community versus hospital care: the crisis in psychiatric provision. Social Science and Medicine 32(4):483–489.

Punukollu NR (1991) Huddersfield (West) Crisis Intervention Team: four years follow-up. Psychiatric Bulletin 15:278–280.

Querido A (1968) The shaping of community mental health care. British Journal of Psychiatry 114:293–302.

Ratna L (1982) Crisis intervention in psychogeriatrics: a two-year follow-up study. British Journal of Psychiatry 141:296–301.

Reid H (1989) Hospitalized psychiatry. In: Brackx A, Grimshaw C (eds) Mental Health Care in Crisis. London: Pluto.

Rogers A, Pilgrim D (1996) Mental Health Policy in Britain. A critical introduction. Basingstoke: Macmillan Press.

Rollin HR (1977) 'De-institutionalization' and the community: fact and theory. Psychological Medicine 7:181–184.

Rubenstein D (1972) Rehospitalization versus family crisis intervention. American Journal of Psychiatry 129(6):715–720.

Sashidharan SP (1994) Psychiatrists fear care in the community (letter). British Medical Journal 308:1236.

Sayce L, Craig TKJ, Boardman AP (1991) The development of community mental health centres in the UK. Social Psychiatry and Psychiatric Epidemiology 26:14–20.

Scull A (1977) Decarceration. Englewood Cliffs, NJ: Prentice-Hall.

Shorter E (1997) A History of Psychiatry From the Era of the Asylum to the Age of Prozac. New York: John Wiley.

Simpson CJ, Seager CP, Robertson JA (1993) Home-based care and standard hospital care for patients with severe mental illness: a randomised controlled trial. British Journal of Psychiatry 162:239–243.

Stein LI, Test MA (1980) Alternative to mental hospital treatment. I. Conceptual model, treatment program, and clinical evaluation. Archives of General Psychiatry 37:392–397.

Stein LI, Test MA, Marx AJ (1975) Alternative to the hospital: a controlled study. American Journal of Psychiatry 132(5):517–522.

Szasz TS (1972) The Myth of Mental Illness. St Albans: Paladin.

Test MA, Stein LI (1980) Alternative to mental hospital treatment: III. Social costs. Archives of General Psychiatry 37:409–412.

Thomas B (1998) Past insights for present problems. Nursing Times 94(17):57–60.

Tyrer P (1995) Essential issues in community psychiatry. In: Tyrer P, Creed F (eds) Community Psychiatry in Action. Analysis and prospects. Cambridge: Cambridge University Press.

Weisbrod BA, Test MA, Stein LI (1980) Alternative to mental hospital treatment II. Economic benefit-cost analysis. Archives of General Psychiatry 37:400–405.

Whittle P, Mitchell S (1997) Community alternatives project: an evaluation of a community-based acute psychiatric team providing alternatives to admission. Journal of Mental Health 6(4):417–427.

CHAPTER 2

Intensive home treatment services: the current position in the UK

SARAH ORME

Summary

Results are presented from a nationwide survey of the provision of crisis, home treatment and other emergency mental health services. The survey process and means of classifying home treatment services are reported. Issues considered include service aims, hours of operation, personnel, the management and supervision of staff and interventions offered to clients.

The survey

This chapter presents results from a nationwide survey of the provision of crisis, home treatment and other emergency services. The survey grew out of an interest in whether those services that had been found through a literature review of published research were still in operation, how many had closed and how many services had developed, but perhaps did not have this level of exposure.

A standard letter was sent to every UK Health Authority or Board (127 authorities in total) between July and December 1997, asking what crisis, home treatment and other emergency mental health services were purchased. The letter also asked for the operational policies for services to be sent to the author if available, or for a contact person within services to be identified who could be contacted for further information. The initial letter was addressed to mental health commissioning and purchasing managers/directors within health authorities as it was assumed they would know what services were being purchased.

To date, a response rate of 89% ($n = 113$) has been achieved from health authorities and boards. Services identified by purchasers have been followed up and operational policies, service specifications, evaluation documents and any other documentation available in the public domain requested. Follow-up letters have since been written to team leaders or other principal personnel for clarification on some issues.

A database has been designed to record all service information. A series of issues have been identified as important to crisis and home treatment service provision (e.g. DoH 1994, 1996, 1998, Stein and Test 1980, Cobb 1995, Minghella et al 1998) and these were considered in compiling the database. For example, whether services were multidisciplinary, whether they offered 24-hour access and interventions, any key worker and care planning arrangements, preferred referring agents and so on were considered for inclusion and recorded.

To date, information from 152 sets of service documentation has been entered into the database, of which 48 services (32%) reported that they offered some sort of home treatment to clients. The other services represented within the database include crisis response teams, out-of-hours telephone lines, crisis beds and crisis centres, to name a few.

Previous studies

Previous surveys of mental health service provision have been carried out, three of which are directly relevant to this work. The Value For Money Unit produced a directory of mental health crisis services in the UK (VFMU 1997). This was compiled following a one-off mailing to all health authorities, health trusts, social services departments and voluntary organisations in the UK, so can be identified as having had greater coverage than the present survey. However, they considered the provision of crisis services using the definition of a service as one:

> . . . provided by any agency, for people with mental health problems which is open outside normal working hours (Monday to Friday 9 a.m. to 5 p.m.) and which seeks to support people in a time of need/crisis. (VFMU 1997)

The classification of services utilised by the VFMU does not easily lend itself to the identification of home treatment services. Briefly, it reports details of 16 crisis helplines, 30 24-hour crisis services (including crisis intervention, crisis response, outreach, psychiatric emergency and home treatment services), 32 non-24-hour crisis services, 11 safe houses/respite accommodation, 18 befriending services and four Accident and Emergency crisis services. Court diversion and crisis card schemes are also reported on. Each service is described on an A4 sheet in terms of the size of population served, length of time the service has been operating, staffing and so on. The directory is a good resource for contacts and basic descriptions of services, but the information contained within it is limited and has not been subject to any comment or analysis.

Another survey is that of Faulkner et al (1994) who carried out a survey of 49 district health authorities to establish the provision of hospital, residential and community support services. The survey took place by telephone in order to maximise response rates, and mental health service managers were targeted as respondents. The survey took place between January and March 1993 and authorities were chosen to represent regional health authorities, with a range of sizes and Jarman UPA scores (indicating levels of social deprivation) across the country, and a balance of urban, rural and mixed areas. Community service provision was considered in terms of crisis intervention teams, continuing care teams for people with long-term mental health problems and residential alternatives to hospital admission. The survey found that three units or trusts (6.5%) had established crisis intervention teams and three (6.5%) had residential alternatives to admission in place. A further five areas (11%) were in the process of considering the development of crisis services. Continuing care teams were more established with 41% of units or trusts having community- or hospital-based teams offering services to those with long-term mental health problems.

Finally, regarding other surveys of mental health service provision, Johnson and Thornicroft (1995) in their survey of emergency mental health services found only 3% of health authorities had staffed 24-hour services.

Limitations of the current study

The limitations of this present survey need to be raised at the outset.

- First, the survey only approached health authorities and boards as purchasers of services, not social services departments. This means some services will have been missed. Also, voluntary organisations and health NHS trusts were not approached and asked what services they provided until identified by a health authority purchaser.

- Second, as with most surveys, the findings rely upon respondents and should be considered in this light. As indicated above, 11% of health authorities have not responded to the initial request for information. Also, a number of trusts have not provided detailed service information after 2 years, despite follow-up requests. The services in the database represent around 80 health authorities, despite responses from 113. Taking into account that 19 authorities reported they did not purchase any crisis or home treatment services, that still leaves a number of authorities that are unrepresented – these are being followed up.

- Finally, a point needs to be made about the duration of this survey and collection of data. It has taken over 2 years to amass the service information contained within the database. Services have been followed up in order to try to fill in any gaps in the information known about them. However, this has not allowed any developments or changes in service provision to be followed up in any systematic way. The author knows the setting up of home treatment services has started in some areas. However, without systematic regular mailings to try to gather information it is not known how far service development has progressed. Therefore changes may have been made to service provision and new services developed that are not reported below.

Bearing in mind all of the above, the present survey suggests that crisis service provision has increased since the survey of Faulkner et al (1994). Despite the fact that both Faulkner et al and the present survey focused on NHS provision and purchasing, it can be seen that many more crisis services are being provided now compared to 1993–94. The Value For Money Unit (VFMU 1997) surveyed much more widely by considering social services and voluntary agencies as providers of services, but still the present survey was able to gather data on a greater number of services. A follow-up survey, in perhaps another 5 years, would be useful to see how service development has continued or indeed changed in emphasis.

Definitions and terminology

An initial problem when considering mental health crisis or home treatment provision is the terminology applied to services. No agreed definition exists as to what an IHT service is, the service components it must contain, or how services should be designed. Suggestions are contained within the home treatment research literature and some UK services can be seen to be based on these models. For example, some UK services have been identified as being based on the training in community living (TCL) or psychiatric assertive community treatment (PACT) model of Stein and Test (1980).

The PACT model is defined as one that includes:

> ... provision of a full range of medical, psychosocial, and rehabilitation services by a community-based team that operates 7 days a week, 24 hours a day. (Burns and Santos 1995, p. 669)

PACT teams must offer core interdisciplinary teams responsible for a fixed group of clients; assertive outreach and *in vivo* treatment in the community; individual treatment with tailor-made interventions; ongoing treatment and support (Taube et al 1990). Burns and Santos (1995) also suggest that the terms PACT, continuous treatment and assertive treatment teams can be used interchangeably. It should be noted, however, that 'assertive treatment' as used here does not necessarily mean the same as UK 'assertive outreach' where services focus on clients considered 'difficult to engage', long-term users of mental health services who require regular monitoring and those who are prone to lose contact with services (DoH 1998).

In general, UK home-based mental health services incorporate some of the above aspects of treatment, but not all, and tend to offer intensive, time-limited care. However, the titles given to UK services are different, in that services use names such as IHT team, home treatment service and community treatment team.

The names of services within the database were not, therefore, taken as an indicator of whether or not a service offered home treatment. Rather the author 'blindly' examined service information for the 48 services that considered themselves to offer home treatment. Without reference to service names, a deductive process was undertaken of reading through service documentation and identifying from this whether or not a service offered home treatment. The definition of an IHT service utilised here was that of Brimblecombe (see Introduction, this volume) and services identified as home treatment if they:

- offered home treatment as an alternative to admission;
- were open for longer than office hours;
- provided a rapid response to those facing admission.

From a database of 152 services, 48 had been identified initially as offering treatment in clients' homes on the basis of information contained within service operational documentation, or following contact with service providers. These 48 services were separated from the full database and then considered, first, in terms of their hours of operation. Fifteen services were excluded from further analysis at this stage: five because insufficient detail on the hours of operation was available; two operated only out of office hours; 2 had ceased operating; and six operated office hours only. These services were excluded because they did not fit the second criterion, that is they did not operate for longer than office hours, or this could not be ascertained from the documentation provided. Another nine services were identified as offering a service distinct from home treatment and two services were considered borderline but were excluded because they could not be identified conclusively as offering home treatment services. This left 22 services that clearly met the definition for an IHT service adopted here (see Table 2.1).

Home treatment service characteristics

Distribution of services

The Department of Health claimed in 1998 that home treatment services were not widespread (DoH 1998). Whether this statement meant in terms of number or geographical location is not clear. If in terms of numbers, it may be considered to be accurate as only one in seven of the services found through the above survey can be identified as offering home treatment services. If, however, one considers the geographical distribution of services, this statement is perhaps more inaccurate. Accepting that this chapter may not be fully

Table 2.1: The 22 services discussed in detail

Service name	Health Authority*	Year started	MDT	24 hours	Source of information
Community Alternatives Project	South and West Devon	1993	Yes	No	Evaluation report
Community Support Team	Borders	?	No	No	Service proposal
Community Support Team	Northumberland	1994	No	No	Service profile
Intensive Home Treatment Team	Leeds	1993	Yes	Yes	Information pack
Home Treatment Service	Lincolnshire	1998	Yes	Yes	Operational policy
Inner City Crisis Team	Avon	1997	Yes	No	Operational policy
Home Treatment Team	Birmingham	1996	Yes	Yes	Operational policy
Psychiatric Acute Community Treatment Team	Avon	1997	No	No	Operational policy
High Peak Intensive Home Support Service	North Derbyshire	1997	Yes	Yes	Operational policy
Intensive Home Nursing Service	Tees	1998	No	No	Operational policy
Mental Health Crisis Assessment & Home Support (Nursing) Team	Gateshead and South Tyneside	1997	No	No	Service profile
Home Option Service	Manchester	1997	Yes	Yes	Information pack
Primary Mental Health Care Team	Manchester	1993	Yes	Yes	Policies and protocols
Home Treatment Service	Bradford	1996	Yes	Yes	Operational policy
South West Assertive Outreach Team	Lothian	?	Yes	No	Operational policy
Home Treatment Service	Brent and Harrow	1998	No	No	Finance application
Community Teams	Buckinghamshire	1984	Yes	No	Operational policy
Home Treatment Service	Birmingham	?	Yes	Yes	Operational policy/guidelines
Mental Health Crisis Service	Liverpool	1996	No	Yes	Operational policy
Rapid Assessment and Home Treatment Service	Northumberland	1991	No	No	Information pack
Intensive Home Treatment Team	North and East Devon	1998	Yes	No	Operational policy
Community Treatment Team	West Hertfordshire	1994	Yes	No	Operational policy

* Please note Health Authority has been included rather than Trust, as Health Authority boundaries seem to change less frequently.

representative of all services (see above), there does seem to be a wide geographical distribution of services.

Home treatment services exist in Scotland (e.g. Borders Community Support Team) and southern England (e.g. Exeter and District Intensive Home Treatment Team). They exist in rural (Northumberland, Derbyshire Dales) and city centre (Manchester, Birmingham) areas. If one looks at a map of the UK in terms of the health authority boundaries, some areas are well served (e.g. Avon, some inner cities) whereas other regions do not appear to have home treatment services (e.g. Wales and Northern Ireland – but a very low response rate was achieved from both these areas). However, as home treatment services are continually being developed in light of government guidelines requiring the development of 24-hour community-based services (DoH 1996, 1998), the picture of home treatment services in the UK is constantly changing and, with the emphasis of the National Service Framework (DoH 1999) again on 24-hour community services, the distribution of IHT services, both in terms of number and geography, can only improve.

A related issue to the distribution of services is the size of populations served by them. Unfortunately this is not very often included in operational documentation and details were available for only seven of the 22 services. Populations served, however, ranged in size from around 57 000 by one team to 230 000 between two teams. City populations covered were around 120 000 (Manchester) to 130 000 (Birmingham, Leeds) with more rural teams offering services to populations ranging from 57 000 to 120 000. Those services catering to mixed rural and urban populations had larger catchment areas serving populations of between 205 000 and 230 000.

Funding

The ways in which services are funded is important in that this may determine the longevity of services. For example, Mental Health Challenge Fund money was initially available for a limited period of 3 years. Of the 22 services here, nine did not report how they were funded in their service documentation. Of the others, four were purchased by health authorities and four funded via joint health and social services budgets. Three had been funded via the Mental Health Challenge Fund, one as a Spectrum of Care Project with social services, and one via a Mental Illness Specific Grant. One service stated they had been offered additional funding through Mental Health Challenge Funds.

Funding arrangements may now have changed, however, in that Mental Health Challenge and Mental Illness Specific Grant funded services may now have been absorbed into health authority recurring budgets; indeed, some services may have ceased operating. Also, changes to the funding of services will occur following the reconfiguration of joint finance initiatives in April 2000.

Longevity

Little can be said about the longevity of services as most of those included here were relatively recent in their inception. Three services did not provide details of when they first started operating. However, of those that did, four services started operating in 1998 and five in 1997. Three were set up in 1996, two in 1994, three in 1993, one in 1991 and one in 1984. It can be seen then that two services have been operating for longer periods than the majority. One of these older services was set up as a project to offer community mental health services to a defined population, and the other developed as a rapid response and home treatment service. Both operate in largely rural areas with outlying villages. It may be that the relative 'newness' of the other services represented is due to the relatively recent calls from government to develop home treatment services (DoH 1994, 1996) and also an example of how long it takes policy to become reality.

Aims of services

Moving on to the operational arrangements for services, service documents were re-examined in order to ascertain the aims and objectives (additional to those identified by Brimblecombe's definition), and, in some cases, the philosophy of services. Seventeen services explicitly stated that they were offered as an alternative to, or in place of, hospital admission; 12 also worked to facilitate early discharge from hospital. Seven services aimed their provision at clients with severe or enduring mental illness and ten at those with acute mental health problems or those in crisis. Seven services aimed to reduce the demand for inpatient admissions or prevent unnecessary admissions; four aimed to reduce lengths of hospital stay. Other services aimed to respond rapidly to those in need (six), to develop follow-up and liaison with community services (four) and to facilitate necessary admissions. Support for users, reducing the risk of relapse and reducing stress-related illnesses in families or informal carers were also objectives of some services.

As can be seen from these aims, the philosophy behind services is mainly psychosocial rather than medical, in that 'cure' or diagnosis-based treatment was not mentioned by any service. The onus is on services to provide care, treatment and support to individuals in their own homes, in some cases involving the client's own social network in this process. The aim of over half the services to facilitate discharge from hospital, by providing clients with support during the transition from hospital to community-based care, is also an aspect of service provision that distinguishes home treatment services from other types of provision and illustrates their psychosocial rather than medical approach to care. Whether these aims can be met by the interventions offered by services will be considered later.

Clients: inclusion and exclusion criteria

The services considered here generally targeted specific clients determined by inclusion and exclusion criteria. Only one service reported that it did not target specific clients; even so, it accepted clients only from the local electoral ward. Three services did not provide any information regarding exclusion criteria and four reported they had no specific exclusion policies.

Clients were targeted in terms of the problems they were experiencing. For example, 15 services focused on clients in crisis or with acute mental health problems or acute mental illness. Nine services were targeted at those suffering severe or enduring mental illness and ten targeted those at risk of, or facing, admission. Exclusions were also expressed in terms of diagnoses and 11 services did not intervene with those who had a primary diagnosis of substance abuse or required detoxification. Six services excluded those with a primary diagnosis of organic brain disorder.

Fifteen services defined target clients in terms of their age: ten offered services to clients aged from 16 to 64 or 65 and three for the age range 18–65. Of the services that included specific exclusion criteria, seven excluded in terms of age; four excluded people under 16, one excluded those under 17 and two excluded people over 65. This shows up the variation throughout the country in the use of definitions regarding child and adolescent, adult, and elderly services. It also suggests that home treatment services are not provided to children or the elderly and raises the question of what services are available for these groups when they are in acute need or crisis as an alternative to hospitalisation.

As well as clients' current problems, risk behaviours were considered as reasons for inclusion or exclusion depending on individual services. For example, a few services targeted clients at risk of relapse, those at risk of suicide and those at risk of self-harm or harm to others. A greater number of services (six) excluded clients considered a risk to others, and risk of suicide or self-harm were also reasons for exclusion of clients from some services.

Additional targeting criteria for clients included residence locally (seven), clients' willingness to cooperate (four) or clients requiring detoxification from alcohol or drugs. Being registered with a local GP, having accommodation, fulfilling specific Care Programme Approach categories and having access to social support were other considerations in accepting clients.

Clients excluded from services included those with learning disabilities, clients whose primary problem was relationship or domestic violence issues, those detained under the Mental Health Act, those non-resident locally, those seeking accommodation or non-compliant; three services were limited by the number of places available to clients.

Coupled to the confusion that may be caused by differences in the age cut-off criteria for some services, is the realisation that some of these services will only deal with known psychiatric clients. The definition of an IHT service adopted here states that services should help clients facing admission and offer an alternative to this. However, this situation may occur for those both known and new to secondary mental health services, whereas nearly half the services here are targeted at clients identified as experiencing severe or enduring problems. The exclusion of new clients from alternatives to hospitalisation is worrying because of the accumulated evidence of problems caused by stays on inpatient wards (Goffman 1961). Indeed, it is perhaps these new clients who might benefit most from a home treatment service preventing them becoming part of the inpatient mental health system.

Requiring clients to meet specific Care Programme Approach criteria highlights that some services are targeted at very specific groups of clients. As each service had its own target and exclusion criteria no generalisations can be made, however, it seems clear that, in the main, services are targeted at known clients (this can be seen again below in the consideration of who is able to refer clients). As with the case for the young and elderly, it must be asked what alternative services to hospitalisation are available for new clients and those with diagnoses that these home treatment services regularly exclude, namely those with drug, alcohol or organic problems.

Referring agents

As well as defining clients in terms of target and exclusion criteria, the clients served by services are also determined in terms of those agencies allowed to refer to services. Three of the 22 services stated that they operated an open referrals policy. However, of these three, only one was open to all, one was open to clients and carers previously known to the service, and one was open to service users only 9 a.m.–5 p.m. Monday to Friday. The 'openness' of these services therefore needs to be considered in light of the policies of other services.

Of the other services, no clear pattern as to whom was able to refer clients emerged. Four services accepted clients only after they had been assessed by the Community Mental Health Team (CMHT) or ward staff. All other services had individual ideas on who acceptable referrers might be. For example, one service accepted referrals from the primary care mental health team, the continuing needs team, the Emergency Duty Team, local hospital, the police, GPs, non-statutory mental health organisations and the assertive outreach team. Another accepted referrals only from the sector consultant.

In some services referring agents were different depending on whether the client was a new referral. For example, GPs and consultants had to refer new referrals, but GPs, consultants, the CMHT or other professionals could refer known clients. In another case a GP referral was required for a new referral, otherwise key workers could refer. Finally, in some cases, a number of different professionals could refer, but a medical assessment had to be completed, for example, a consultant, CPN or social worker could refer clients, but a medical assessment had to be completed before clients were accepted into the service.

With the emphasis on referrals following assessment by mental health professionals, gatekeeping access to services can be seen to be an important role fulfilled by these referral procedures.

Hours of operation

Funding and resources will have an impact on when services are available. This in turn may affect the ability of services to deliver care to clients. The 22 services included here are already known to offer services outside office hours. Further consideration was given to the reported hours of operation to see if any predominant model of opening hours existed.

Eight services claimed to offer a 24-hour service; however, of these, seven operated an on-call service at some point during the day. For example, one operated on an on-call basis from 5 p.m. to 9 a.m. seven days a week, and another offered a 24-hour on-call service for all clients accepted by the team. Only one service reported that it operated throughout the 24-hour period without using any on-call staff.

Of the remaining 14 services, five operated from 9 a.m. until 9 p.m., seven days a week. Others offered a mixture of extended hours Monday–Friday and limited operating at weekends. In total 13 services operated for 11–14 hours Monday–Friday with a variety of opening times over weekends and bank holidays.

It can be seen that these types of service do offer care and support for clients outside the normal office hours of 9 a.m.–5 p.m. However, 24-hour staffed services are still rare and on-call arrangements vary across services. For example, the number of staff and disciplines available out-of-hours, whether they are working from a base or their own homes and whether visiting is carried out alone or jointly, will affect the services that can be offered to clients. Also, weekend working is still limited in many cases to office hours or less. A few services stated that they worked flexibly around their defined hours, but this still raises the question of what happens to clients if they experience a crisis when the service is not available.

Staffing

The staffing reported within service operational documentation was examined to ascertain the disciplines offering services to clients and the grades or skill-mix of staff within services. Eight services were unidisciplinary – seven were nursing only (although three had sessional input from psychiatrists), and one was offered by social services staff only.

Fourteen services were therefore multidisciplinary. Of these 14, all included nursing staff. Four services were operated by nurses and psychiatrists, two by nurses and occupational therapists, two by nurses and social work staff. Others had varying mixes of nurses, psychiatrists, social workers, psychologists and occupational therapists. One service employed an ex-service user in a service development role.

Role responsibility was not described in detail within service protocols. The interventions offered by services (see below) were described, but without stipulating which disciplines carried out which tasks or whether staff adopted a generic role within teams. The numbers and grades of staff were reported in some cases and this is described below. Six services did not include details of the number or grading of staff. The number of staff in the other 16 services ranged from 21 to three.

As has already been stated, all those services providing details of staff disciplines bar one included nursing as a key discipline in providing care. Of these, however, the mix between qualified (H–E grades) and unqualified (A–B) grades varied.

Two services included H grade nurses – one as a manager, one in an unspecified role. In all teams there was a greater number of qualified staff than unqualified ones. Nursing teams ranged from 18 RMNs (no grades specified) to one of 4.5 qualified and one unqualified nursing staff. Another team had 11 qualified nurses, three unqualified ones, three occupational therapists (one Senior I OT, two Senior II OTs) with psychiatry input. Where sufficient detail was available the ratio between qualified and unqualified was calculated. Staffing ratios of qualified to unqualified staff ranged from 14 : 3 in two cases, to 4 : 2 in three cases.

The largest team consisted of 21 members, excluding clerical and administration staff, and the smallest 3. Six teams ranged from 17 to 21 staff members and seven teams had six staff or less; three teams consisted of 8–10.5 staff.

As with referral policies for services there is great variation in the staffing component of these home treatment teams. This does not seem to be driven by population size, although the number of services that provided details of both sizes of team and population is very small and generalisations cannot be made from these numbers.

Additional details on the clients actually seen by services, and when, may account for staff make-up – this detail is not available in service operational documents but may be made clear through service audit processes. All that can be said for the moment is that there is great variation across teams and, as with the hours of operation of services, this may greatly affect the interventions that can be offered to clients.

Training, management and supervision

Coupled to staffing are the issues of training, management and supervision of staff. Details of these were not always included in service documentation, and in most cases efforts have been made to follow up services individually in order to ascertain this information. However, lack of response from some services ensures that this information remains incomplete. Even so, it can be seen that in each of these three areas, practice within services is highly different.

Training

Training was examined in terms of whether staff received additional or service-specific training prior to working in home treatment services. Six services provided no additional information on training; one stated that the locality manager was looking into suitable training options and another stated no additional training had been offered to staff. Other services provided highly individualised responses such that verbatim reports are reproduced below.

One service offered staff training in cognitive behavioural, problem solving and communication skills. Staff members were also trained to help carers and/or clients identify early warning signs of illness. Another service offered a 2-week induction programme composed of speakers from established services, risk training, personal safety training and writing the service operational policy. In one service induction was followed by training in behavioural family therapy and the use of outcome measures. Other services offered training in the core competencies of risk assessment, care planning, psychosocial training and the Mental Health Act, as well as introductory counselling.

These examples show where specific training programmes were available. In other services less specific training was on offer. For example, one offered health and safety training (basic life support, manual handling, etc.) and stated that it was the responsibility of team members to engage in continuous professional and service development. Other staff were offered alternate weekly sessions to update them on issues relevant to their work; mandatory training courses dealt with violence and restraint. In another service, following induction, staff members were to keep up to date with current developments and offered training in evidence-based treatment. Even more nebulous responses included: relevant ongoing training; ongoing professional and personal development; access to training as appropriate; some training sessions offered on an ad hoc basis.

It can be seen from all of the above that training for staff offering home treatment services is by no means standardised. Indeed in some cases there is no specific training and in others it is up to individual staff members to ensure that their training needs are addressed, for example by keeping abreast of new developments in the field. Bearing in mind the different disciplines from which staff members in some teams are drawn, the different philosophies that exist within these disciplines, and well-documented problems experienced by some multidisciplinary teams (Practices made Perfect 1997), it is surprising that more teams did not offer team-building opportunities. This could, however, be accounted for by nearly half the teams being staffed solely by nurses, with or without psychiatric input. This issue is another that affects staff ability to serve clients and needs greater consideration in service development.

Management

As with training, management arrangements were peculiar to services. Eleven services did not provide any detailed information and, of the others, no two services had similar arrangements. In the simplest of cases, a team manager was accountable to the acute services manager.

In other cases the responsibility for line management and for the day-to-day running of services were separated. For example, in one service the clinical team leader had line management responsibility for nurses and occupational therapists and the team co-ordinator was responsible for the day-to-day running of the team. In another the team manager managed the day-to-day running of the service but a senior clinical nurse had line management responsibility for nurses and unqualified staff.

Where multidisciplinary teams existed, management often depended on the discipline of staff members. For example, in one team administration, nursing, psychology and occupational therapy staff were managerially accountable to the service leader who in turn was accountable to the NHS trust community services manager, whereas the care manager, social workers and rehabilitation officer were accountable through the social services management structure. Medical staff within this team had yet another management structure: consultant medical staff were managerially accountable to the chief executive and junior doctors to their consultant. This separation of management in terms of discipline was repeated elsewhere and in five services health and social services staff were managed separately within their own discipline.

This latter finding is of particular relevance bearing in mind the National Service Framework (DoH 1999) commitment to developing single management structures for multidisciplinary services. It can be seen that much more work may be required before this is the common practice. The above also highlights variation in the use of terminology within mental health services, this time within trusts when describing similar management roles and responsibilities.

Supervision

Again, as with training and management of staff, supervision arrangements were often individual to each service. Eight services did not report any supervision arrangements. In the other services supervision arrangements were not always clear. As with training, some services were specific as to when, and how much, supervision should take place. For example, one service stated that team members were expected to have at least 1 hour of clinical supervision a month, but that it was the individual's and their professional advisor's responsibility to ensure that clinical supervision took place. Elsewhere professional supervision was to be provided by someone of the same discipline and clinical supervision provided at least once every 3 weeks. Another service described how group supervision was available monthly from someone external to the team and individual supervision should take place for 2 hours at least twice a month. More than one service stated that supervision was available during team meetings and at daily handovers.

The variation in practice between teams can again be seen. In all these three areas, training, management and supervision, large differences in teams were apparent, which may be a reflection of different team make-up and service organisation. However, these three issues – training, management and supervision – taken with the differences in staffing arrangements may have an effect on staff morale and the capability and confidence staff feel they have to do their job, which again may affect the ability of services to help clients.

Interventions

All of the above issues in some way impinge on the interventions offered to clients. In particular, staffing of services in terms of disciplines, grades and training in specific skills or therapies will have a large effect on what services can actually do with, and for, clients. The interventions offered to clients detailed in service documents (information was sparse in some cases) were classified for ease of comparison and frequency of stated interventions reported. The majority of services assessed clients (15) and drew up care plans (12) based on client need or the needs of their social support network (14). Carers and families of clients were supported by services (14), mental state was monitored (5) and ongoing support offered by some (2). Services also monitored and/or administered medication (10), provided education on mental health issues to clients and their carers (10), offered problem-solving or adaptive coping skills training (8), offered practical help (8) and help with activities of daily living (6).

Specific interventions offered by teams included cognitive behavioural therapy, family therapy, short-term counselling, anxiety and stress management, and social and leisure activities. Only one service mentioned that they used complementary therapies with clients. In order to ensure continuity of care, 11 services liaised with colleagues to ensure acute or longer-term care was offered to clients when required. Other services offered respite facilities or were able to refer clients on to other services for specific treatment or therapy.

The Care Programme Approach

Sixteen services stated that they were integrated with the Care Programme Approach (CPA) or offered services to clients within this system of care; six services did not provide any information. Three services also offered services to clients under the social services care management programme, although 17 services reported no details and two stated they were not involved with it. Again, with the integration of these two forms of case management (see NHS Executive/Social Services Inspectorate 1999), changes may have since occurred in service provision.

Key worker arrangements varied, with six home treatment services taking on the role of CPA key worker, whereas another six services stated that this role remained with the local CMHT or multidisciplinary team (MDT). Eight services offered home treatment named workers in addition to CPA key workers who remained outside the service. Two services provided no details regarding key worker input.

Continuity of care

Continuity of care is operationalised here as continuity across different services and agencies in order to ensure that clients receive services in a continuous and unbroken manner from someone (see Johnson et al 1997 for a discussion of additional definitions of continuity of care). Specific questions were asked regarding interventions to ensure continuity of care: in particular, whether or not home treatment services referred clients on to other services, fed back the outcomes of care to referring agents or clients' GPs, offered discharge planning, or were closely linked to local services.

Sixteen services stated that they referred clients on to other services; six provided no information. Of those that did refer on, in some cases this was if the home treatment service was felt to be inappropriate. Other services referred clients to specialist services dependent on client need, on to appropriate agencies prior to discharge, or back to existing services or their care co-ordinator. Clients were also referred to CMHTs and other services for long-term care.

Regarding feedback, 18 services said they provided feedback and four provided no information on this issue. Feedback processes included a discharge summary being sent to the referrer on discharge, or feedback to GPs, key workers and other agencies informing them of the aftercare plans for clients or of significant clinical outcomes. In some cases the GP was sent details of the key worker and care plan via a standard form; the key worker then informed the GP of referral back to mainstream services and of suggestions for further management and/or early warning signs.

Discharge planning was reported to take place in 14 services and not reported in eight. Discharge planning was implemented by some services in order to create a smooth transition of care between services and encourage continuity of care. In some cases, discharge planning began immediately clients became involved with the home treatment service through identifying agencies to follow-up clients. Other examples of discharge planning included:

- prioritisation of transfers from home treatment services to the CMHT in order to facilitate throughput of clients from acute services
- agreeing aftercare arrangements for clients across agencies
- discharge taking place following a joint decision between the client, team and key worker that there had been a resolution of the presenting problem.

Finally, whether or not services were closely integrated with other services was considered. Twenty-one services reported close liaison with other services; only one did not. Another service felt that close liaison would ensure that the home treatment service enhanced rather than duplicated current service provision. One described close communication with referring agents and GPs throughout the clients' treatment. Other services were closely integrated with local community mental health services or sector teams, held regular meetings with ward staff or aimed to be fully integrated with community and hospital mental health services to improve continuity of care.

To summarise, the interventions offered to clients seem to be less variable across the different services than other areas of service provision. Assessment, care planning and consideration of the needs of clients and their social network were offered by the majority of services. More differentiation was found when one considered specific issues such as the implementation of the CPA, key worker and discharge planning arrangements. When one reconsiders the principal aims of services, that is to offer an alternative to hospital admission, to facilitate earlier discharge from hospital, to offer support to clients and their carers and to adopt a psychosocial approach, then it can be argued that the interventions presented here should enable services to achieve these goals.

Average length of contact

Briefly, a final few issues that were identified within service documentation are reported. Length of contact may be determined both in advance of a client coming into contact with a service or determined during the client's contact. Six services offered no information on the preferred or actual length of contact with clients, but a number of services had carried out internal or external evaluations and calculated the average length of time for which clients were in contact with services. As with other service design issues discussed above, this was another area where much variation was found.

Mean lengths of stay, calculated from evaluation studies, ranged from 16 days to 8.5 weeks with two services reporting calculated averages of 22 days and 32 days. One service evaluation distinguished between the length of time spent with clients accepted into the service in order to facilitate discharge and those offered home treatment as an alternative to admission. Clients offered an alternative to admission were in contact for nearly 2 weeks longer, on average, than those leaving hospital early. Other home treatment teams stipulated in advance (in their operational policies) the length of time for which a service was offered. One offered services for as long as required dependent on clinical need.

Broadly speaking services can be split into those that offer treatment for a month or less (seven services) or over a month (seven); however, it must be remembered that there is much variation across the different services. Also, the preferred length of contact with clients defined in operational documentation may differ from that actually experienced by service users dependent on their needs. This would need to be investigated by a comparison of planned and actual length of contacts and was beyond the scope of this study. Bearing in mind what has been said about the similarity in the interventions offered, it is interesting to note the variation in the duration for which these interventions may be offered.

Staff safety

Staff safety was initially considered in terms of whether written policies existed for staff carrying out visits to clients' homes, although some services referred to safety on service premises. Whether or not service documentation included details of a staff safety policy was recorded. In eight cases there was no information about safety within service documentation. In three cases a detailed policy was available separately, but in 11 cases the service description included details. As with other issues, safety policies varied quite widely and three examples are presented here.

One service stated that on-call nurse visits were normally carried out alone, but that the on-call nurse could take the second on-call nurse with them at their discretion. Otherwise the on-call nurse should inform their spouse of where they were going and when they intended to return. In another case, staff carried mobile phones, worked in pairs where necessary, kept diaries up to date and notified colleagues before and after visiting clients in uncertain risk circumstances. Finally, in one case the acute admission ward was given details of each out-of-hours call, including the name and address of the client. If a staff member did not contact ward staff at a pre-arranged time then the ward staff attempted to contact the home treatment staff member. If there was no response, then the police were informed of the situation.

Only three examples are cited here but, even so, much variation can be seen with this small number. If one predominant model of staff safety policy did exist, it was based on the latter example above. In a number of cases staff reported where they were going, arranged a time to contact services or estimated when they would return and action was taken if this contact did not take place. The personnel to be contacted in this event, and how many procedures were completed prior to contacting the police, were where most services varied in their approach.

Overall model of home treatment in the UK

An important question for the author to address in this chapter was: does the existence of IHT services suggest a general theoretical model based on the need for these services? Unfortunately, the need for these services in particular areas, or decisions made as to service development, are not addressed in service documentation. It is known that in some areas, crisis services have been developed in response to user demands, but this is not evident from the information provided here regarding home treatment services. Leaving aside the need for services, the question asks whether there is a general theoretical model of services. The answer to this is both yes and no:

yes in terms of the aims of services and interventions offered to clients; no in terms of individual service design.

The use of Brimblecombe's definition of IHT services restricted the number of services identified as offering home treatment. The exclusion of certain services may have ensured that certain aspects of service delivery were found to be the same in this analysis. However, it will be noted that great variation was found across the 22 services included in terms of their design and delivery of specific aspects of care. Consideration of the borderline and additional services excluded from this review due to the definition adopted may have provided a broader picture of the type of home treatment services in this country. However, it is suggested that their inclusion would only have resulted in more examples of specific service design and not added to the overall model of services.

If we look at the information presented above, which has been taken from services' own documentation, it is easy to think that there is no predominant model of home treatment service provision in the UK today. Despite the fact of much variation across services, there are however some characteristics common to services. For example, if we consider operating hours, most services are staffed for 12 or more hours a day and at least one-third offer on-call provision to cover the 24-hour period. When considering staffing, the majority of services were multidisciplinary and all but one were primarily based on nursing teams. The aim of services to offer an alternative to hospitalisation and facilitate early discharge from hospital was held by over half of the services, and interventions to address these goals were in place for most of the services. Differences occurred in the minutiae of service delivery, that is, in the adapting of services to local circumstances, local mental health service provision and local need in terms of clients, referral policies, staffing and training and communication arrangements.

Adaptation of services to local need has been considered by Goss and Gluckman (1996) who suggested that it is important for purchasers of mental health services to find out what services work in other places and learn from the experiences of other purchasers and providers. However, what works in one area may not do so elsewhere and the wholesale transfer of one service model to another area does not take account of local circumstances and historical and cultural differences. Goss and Gluckman emphasised the need to parcel out the elements of service provision that are transferable from those that are not. It may be this process that accounts for the variation in home treatment service provision found above in terms of service design but not so much in operation.

Phelan, Strathdee and Thornicroft (1995) similarly suggested that successful service development is dependent on strategic planning and must be based on the assessment of local population need: no universal model of service provision can be applied everywhere. Again, adoption of this principle would in part explain the differences in service design noted above. However, as has already been stated, the completion of needs assessment exercises and reasons for service development were not available within service documentation so conclusions about these processes cannot be made.

Conclusion

In total, 22 services out of a possible 152 were identified that met the definition for an IHT service of operating longer than normal office hours, offering a rapid response and an alternative service to those facing admission. It can be said that using this fairly restrictive definition of IHT identified a relatively small number of services. However, a wide geographical spread of services with different structures, using a variety of names, designed in a number of different ways, but relying on common ways to help clients was identified through this survey. Services called home treatment and community treatment services were found. Both uni- and multidisciplinary teams, operating for between 12 and 24 hours, with a variety of referral policies and exclusion criteria were identified. Despite the variation in service design, it is suggested that a theoretical underpinning of services exists that determines that services offer consistent and similar interventions for clients, even if the length of time for which they do so again varies considerably.

There is likely to be a marked increase in the number of home treatment services over the next few years bearing in mind the emphasis placed on home treatment and community services in the National Service Framework (DoH 1999). It will be interesting to revisit the provision of home treatment in, say, 5 years' time, to ascertain whether similar findings of the variation in design coupled with commonalities of purpose and intervention still exist.

References

Burns BJ, Santos AB (1995) Assertive community treatment: an update of randomized trials. Psychiatric Services 46:669–675.

Cobb A (1995) Community crisis services cost less than hospital care. Open Mind 73:8.

DoH (1994) The Health of The Nation. Key Area Handbook. Mental Illness, 2nd edn. London: HMSO.

DoH (1996) Spectrum of Care. London: HMSO.

DoH (1998) Modernising Mental Health Services. Safe, sound, supportive. London: HMSO.

DoH (1999) A National Service Framework for Mental Health. London: HMSO.

Faulkner A, Field V, Muijen M (1994) A Survey of Adult Mental Health Services. London: Sainsbury Centre for Mental Health.

Goffman E (1961) Asylums: Essays on the Social Situation of Mental Patients and other Inmates. Harmondsworth: Penguin.

Goss T, Gluckman P (1996) Developing a mental health focus for purchasers. In: Thornicroft G, Strathdee G, Commissioning Mental Health Services. London: HMSO.

Johnson S, Thornicroft G (1995) Emergency psychiatric services in England and Wales. British Medical Journal 311:287–288.

Johnson S, Prosser D, Bindman J, Szmukler G (1997) Continuity of care for the severely mentally ill: concepts and measures. Social Psychiatry and Psychiatric Epidemiology 32:137–142.

Minghella E, Ford R, Freeman T, Hoult J, McGlynn P (1998) Open All Hours. London: Sainsbury Centre for Mental Health.

NHS Executive/Social Services Inspectorate (1999) Effective Care Co-ordination in Mental Health Service. Modernising the Care Programme Approach. London: DoH.

Phelan M, Strathdee G, Thornicroft G (1995) The future of mental health emergency services. In: Phelan M, Strathdee G, Thornicroft G, Emergency Mental Health Services in the Community. Cambridge: Cambridge University Press.

Practices made Perfect (1997) Providing Therapists' Expertise in the New NHS: Developing a strategic framework for good patient care. Brighton: Practices made Perfect Ltd.

Stein I, Test MA (1980) Alternative to mental hospital treatment. I. Conceptual model, treatment program, and clinical evaluation. Archives of General Psychiatry 37:392–397.

Taube CA, Morlock L, Burns BA, Santos AB (1990) New directions in research on assertive community treatment. Hospital and Community Psychiatry 41:642–647.

VFMU (1997) Mental Health Crisis Services Directory. Cardiff: Value For Money Unit.

CHAPTER 3

Researching services providing IHT as an alternative to admission

SARAH ORME AND BRUCE COHEN

Summary

Previous approaches to researching home treatment services are considered and problems with these research methodologies addressed. Issues important to general mental health evaluations, as well as specific problems in home treatment research, are described. Suggestions are made regarding future research.

This chapter considers research into home treatment as an alternative to hospital admission as a whole, taking into account the variations and changes in what has constituted such services over the years and in different countries. Consideration of the wide range of topics arising cannot be comprehensive in the limited space available, but an attempt is made to focus on those issues particularly significant in considering both past and future research.

General issues in mental health research

Evaluation is seen as an essential part of any service but is particularly important in the establishment of new services. Evaluations can tell us much more than whether a service is simply 'good' or 'bad': it can assess process and outcome, it can discover otherwise unknown consequences of the programme, it can point to further developments or possible shortcomings to be rectified, and it can help the development of an 'efficient' and 'effective' service (more on these terms later in the chapter). In terms of health service evaluations, research knowledge is very much linked to action, and the scientific model of investigation (i.e. the 'hypo-deductive method') is used to assess the efficiency (or otherwise) of service practices. Health service evaluations aim to 'produce reliable and valid research data on which to base appropriate, effective, cost-effective, efficient and acceptable health services at the primary and secondary care levels' (Bowling 1997, p. 6). Health service evaluations can take many different forms in practice, but usually conform to one of two typical models: 'formative' evaluations, which collect research data whilst the programme or service is in action with the aim of developing or improving it, and 'summative' evaluations, which collect information on the service to decide whether the programme should continue or even be extended. For both types of evaluation of health services and programmes, data is usually collected which pertains to the structure, inputs, processes, outputs and outcomes of the service (Donabedian 1980, cited in Bowling 1997).

As well as health service evaluations being informed primarily by the scientific enterprise of medicine and the medical model of investigation, there is a strong historical link with epidemiology, and the use of statistics from local populations (three historical examples being Booth in London, Rowntree in York, and Engels in Manchester) to make generalised statements about the health needs of the general population.

However, the introduction of consumer choice and patient satisfaction has changed this approach to evaluation somewhat. A 'biopsychosocial model' of ill health advocates assessment of physical, psychological and social events together in assessing the outcomes of a programme. Thus, it is argued that each of these elements needs to be measured in relation to the patient's perceived health status and health-related quality of life, plus the reduction of symptoms and toxicity, as well as the patient's (and carer's, if applicable) satisfaction with the treatment and outcomes (Bowling 1997, p. 13).

Within medicine, 'evaluation' usually means taking a rigid hypo-deductive method of research, such as carrying out randomised controlled trials (RCTs) on new pharmacological compounds or other biochemical methods of medical science. This model expands into the evaluation of medical-based services and service users, where the quantitative methodologies of questionnaires and surveys are most readily used. These can be very useful, especially in large scale sample research, but they can also limit responses and be partial to medicine's political agenda. These issues therefore need to be borne in mind in the consideration of the research presented below and are returned to later in the chapter.

Previous and current approaches to home treatment research

Since the development of Querido's (1968) home-based service in the 1930s for the mentally ill and the finding that many could be treated without the need for hospitalisation, the agenda for the evaluation of subsequent home treatment projects has been consistent. That is to say, evaluations of home-based treatment have been largely concerned with measuring reductions in hospital bed usage and other variables that measure the service as an 'effective alternative' to hospital. The agenda was further defined in the 1960s as comparing control (hospital) and experimental (home treatment) groups of patients in order to evaluate the usefulness of home-based treatment programmes.

Through extensive reviews of these 'alternatives' to hospital (see Braun et al 1981, Kiesler 1982) criticism has been made regarding the lack of uniformity of these comparative trials, rather than of the overall methodology producing such results. As is usually the case with medical science, it was felt that in order to reach fundamental conclusions about whether such projects 'worked', further refinement of the quantitative methodology was required along with further controlling of interfering variables. The legacy of randomised controlled trials can be seen in the major examples of home treatment evaluations from different countries: Stein and Test's (1978) study of their 'Training in Community Living' programme in the US, which was refined by Hoult et al (1983) in their community treatment team in Australia. This model of care was subsequently tried in India by Pai and Kapur (1983), and in the UK by Muijen et al (1992). The methodology involved will be briefly outlined and then some general issues around evaluating home treatment projects will be discussed.

Training in Community Living programme, Wisconsin, US

Stein et al (1975) described a programme of care known as Training in Community Living (TCL). Patients needing admission to hospital were randomly assigned to either standard hospital and aftercare or to the experimental treatment programme, which used specially trained staff to promote daily activities in the community. A total of 65 people were allocated to each group. Outcome measures showed significant differences in ratings of global symptomatology, and six out of ten components of clinical assessment favoured the experimental group at 1 year. The results also showed that the experimental group spent significantly more time living in independent settings, in sheltered employment and in full-time competitive (i.e. open) employment, and scored higher on a self-rated scale of satisfaction with their life situations.

In subsequent papers (see Test and Stein 1980, Weisbrod et al 1980) analysis was carried out of the 'social costs', and economic costs and benefits of both groups. Using a Family Burden Scale administered to the patients' most closely related significant other (e.g. family, friends, official agencies and other professionals) at 1 and 4 months after the patients' admission to either project, it was found that there was no more burden experienced by the families of clients in either group. Likewise, an assessment of arrests, suicidal gestures and use of Emergency Rooms was also carried out and similar results were found in terms of 'community burden'. The large amount of support provided to patients, families and the community by the members in the experimental team was emphasised in accounting for these findings. Finally, Weisbrod et al considered all the benefits and costs they were able to derive in economic terms. The experimental programme was found to have both additional costs and benefits compared with the standard treatment. The researchers concluded that the added benefits of the TCL programme of $1200 per patient per year were nearly $400 more per patient per year than the added costs.

Community Treatment, Sydney, Australia

A similar alternative to hospital was evaluated in Australia (Hoult et al 1983) with similar objectives to Test and Stein, namely:

- to demonstrate the feasibility of treating psychiatric patients in the community as an alternative to hospital admission
- to show this could be done without detriment to the patient, family or community

- to demonstrate that such treatment is no more expensive than standard hospitalisation and aftercare.

Patients presenting for admission were randomly allocated to the experimental or a hospital (control) group. The experimental group received medication, support and counselling, training in basic living and social skills, as well as family intervention, support and education. The community treatment team consisted of eight members, including psychiatric nurses, social workers, occupational therapists, a psychiatrist and a psychologist. Evaluation was carried out at admission, and at 1, 4, 8 and 12 months, by an independent research psychologist.

Questionnaires were administered to patients to measure socio-demographic and medical background, perceptions of current symptoms, difficulties, progress and satisfaction with the treatment received. Questionnaires were also administered to relatives to measure burden, opinions of patients' problems, symptoms and progress, and levels of satisfaction with the particular treatment. Clinical instruments were used to measure patients' mental status (Present State Examination: PSE), psychiatric diagnosis (Brief Psychiatric Rating Scale: BPRS), and patients' overall functioning (Health Sick Rating: HSR). Records were also kept of legal detentions or admissions to other hospitals. A cost analysis was carried out of the two programmes by two economists using objective sources (e.g. hospital records and accounts). The results of the programme showed no increased burden upon the family or community, and it was considered to be significantly more satisfactory and helpful by patients and their relatives. The community treatment achieved better clinical outcomes and cost less than standard hospital care with aftercare.

Home Care Treatment, Bangalore, India

Patients suffering a first episode of mental illness and diagnosed with schizophrenia were alternately assigned to either psychiatric wards with aftercare or to a home care treatment programme (Pai and Kapur 1983). A total of 27 in each group were compared and reported upon. Assessment of clinical status was measured via the BPRS and a number of social functioning scales. A semi-structured interview schedule was designed to assess burden on patients' families, and monetary costs of home care versus hospital treatment were assessed during the 6 month follow-up period. Clinical assessments were carried out eight times during the 6 month follow-up period. Socio-demographic information on each patient was also obtained. The results of the study revealed that the experimental group had better clinical outcomes, better social functioning, and reduced burden on the patients' families. The programme of home care was also found to be more economical.

Daily Living Programme, London, UK

The Daily Living Programme (DLP: Muijen et al 1992, Knapp et al 1994) attempted to build on this successful work. It was the first attempt to replicate such a study of home care in Britain, offering a systematic form of training to patients and staff of the experimental programme, which ran for 3 years. The DLP allowed patients to function at home despite their crises with a minimum of inpatient care, and with the aid of 'assertive outreach' as long as was required by the patient. Intensity and type of care were tailored to individual patient needs. Like the projects already mentioned, the DLP offered a full range of services including 24-hour, 7-days-a-week care, treatment at the site of breakdown, case management, problem-oriented care, help with maintenance or acquisition of daily living skills, support and education of patients' significant others, and advocacy for patients, individually and as a group. The control group were given standard hospital and aftercare.

Clients were assessed at admission to the programme, and at three subsequent times over a 20-month period. A number of different standardised clinical rating scales were utilised for measures of symptomatology, social functioning and social adaptation, which were completed by a number of different psychiatrists. Outcomes were superior for home-based care, with clients scoring slightly better on improved symptoms and social adjustment, and with enhanced patient and relative satisfaction. Most DLP clients were admitted at some point, although lengths of stay were lower. The number of deaths from self-harm were higher in the DLP group, three compared with two in the hospital care group. More tellingly, the researchers report that beyond 20 months, most gains were lost apart from patient and relative satisfaction, with many patients still suffering severe symptoms, poor social adjustment, having no job, and in need of assertive follow-up with heavy staff input.

Further home treatment service evaluations

Variations on the home-based treatment alternative have been piloted elsewhere, though the Test and Stein programme and evaluation remains the benchmark by which success or otherwise of programmes is measured. Very similar programmes were developed and evaluated in Canada by Coates et al (1976) and Fenton et al (1979), with the latter carrying out a 2-year follow-up of home treatment patients. Early randomised controlled trials of home care that did not involve a specific team, but relied on CPN visits (for example see Pasamanick et al 1967, Davis et al 1974), as well as other randomised controlled trials (see Langsley et al 1969, Polak et al 1976, Polak 1978), and controlled non-randomised trials (for instance Grad et al 1968, Mosher et al 1975, 1978) have shown that outcomes of home-based experimental groups are usually superior to the control groups. More recently, UK studies of home-based services have been evaluated in both controlled (Minghella et al 1998) and more descriptive (Whittle and Mitchell 1997) ways. Both studies reported benefits for home treatment over standard care options in terms of reduced cost and reduced bed usage. Minghella et al reported similar levels of symptomatic improvement between home treatment and standard care groups (measured by changes in BPRS score), whereas Whittle and Mitchell sought referrers' opinions of the service, the majority of whom responded that they would recommend the service to a colleague.

The quality of home treatment research

Braun et al (1981), in a review of alternatives to hospital treatment, remarked that many of the studies they reviewed were compromised by shortcomings in design and performance, that is, there were problems with the internal validity of the studies and, as a result, their findings could not be generalised due to the limited selection of the patient populations. Braun et al were quite clear that alternatives to hospital need proper evaluation and should conform to 'generally accepted scientific standards with regard to research design, conduct of investigation, and clarity of writing' (1981, p. 739). Braun et al continued that these evaluations should preferably be randomised controlled studies; however, other reviews of home-based treatment alternatives to hospital care have questioned this. Kiesler (1982) and Uchtenhagen (1986) have stated there are too many independent variables to be able to adequately control such studies. For instance, the outcomes of successful studies like that of Hoult et al (1983) may be due to a range of factors including the client being at home, being 'intensively' treated by staff, the medication provided, relatives' care at home, a mix of these factors, or maybe other 'hidden' variables yet to be discovered (such as personal self-coping strategies for instance).

Other approaches

Though home treatment evaluations still very much conform to previously used quantitative indicators for their success, the positive results of earlier studies (for example Test and Stein 1980, Hoult et al 1983, Muijen et al 1992) have allowed for some flexibility in carrying out additional qualitative research on users, carers and teams of professionals (see for example Hogan et al 1997). Additionally, rather than being simply 'pilot' or 'temporary' projects for experimental testing purposes, some home treatment services have been set up as fully operational alternatives to hospital with evaluation acting as an important part of the service's development (for example Sashidharan and Smyth 1992, Dean et al 1993). These evaluations have 'formative' as well as 'summative' elements to them. In other areas, some health services have created a completely integrated network of community care services for the mentally ill that all but replace hospital care, and include home treatment services within them (see for example Pigott and Trott 1993, Burti and Tansella 1996). In these programmes of care RCTs do not take place, rather the 'experimental groups' that receive home treatment are compared with groups of hospital users from another city location or another part of the country where they have no home treatment service.

More importantly, recent evaluations have attempted to assess other parts of the treatment process beyond the statistical profiling of participants and have pointed to some significant difficulties within the services. For example, both Godfrey and Townsend (1995) and Hogan et al (1997) found from their respective evaluations of crisis services in Leeds and Walsall that these services were acting as support services to hospital rather than an alternative to it. Thus both projects were failing on the important issues of reducing the use of hospital beds and, consequently, of being cost-effective. Through interviews with professionals and managers involved in the setting up of the Walsall service, as well as those involved directly in service delivery, Hogan et al found that protocols of referral were not always followed, none of the staff within the service were trained in crisis techniques, overall the service was not valued as an alternative to hospital by fellow health professionals, and the aims and objectives of the programme had not been stated clearly enough. Godfrey and Townsend carried out in-depth interviews with users and carers of the Intensive Home Treatment Service in Leeds and found that many users had been 'discharged early' to the service from hospital, and stayed in the service for a very long time (an average of two months). Furthermore, 25% of users found the service unreliable in some respects (e.g. workers late to, or missing, appointments). Carers appreciated the service but were concerned that it ignored their own needs for support and dealing with the knock-on effects of illness. Also, in the case of users with severe psychosis, workers often felt unable to 'engage' with these clients.

These evaluations are valuable in that they give indications of just how and why some home treatment services can fail. This information may well have been missed by the more standard monitoring procedures imposed on some project evaluations. Hogan (1997) notes that such evaluations need to move from an 'accounting' approach to a 'continuous' approach of service enhancement, 'in which crisis care is evaluated in the context of the mental health services provision as a whole' (1997, p. 1).

Can community care 'enthusiasts' objectively research IHT services?

It has been suggested that the staffing of home treatment teams may account for the positive outcomes of research studies. This may occur in two ways.

- Firstly, Dedman (1993) suggested that studies recruit motivated staff who may differ in their attitudes from staff in the routine services with which research projects are compared. Tyrer (1995a) added that a related issue is the cohesiveness of the staff in teams and that a team operating with a common purpose and philosophy will work better than one that is fragmented, and hence service outcomes will be affected. Staff attitudes and working relationships may therefore affect outcomes.

- Secondly, and perhaps more worrying, is the suggestion that researchers in home treatment services may be biased. Coid (1994, p. 806) asks '. . . can those who so strongly espouse the community-based approach, and who stand to gain most from its implementation, objectively evaluate their own services'. Murray (reported in Tyrer 1995b) stated that he knew of no research in community care that compared an enthusiast-run service with a non-enthusiast-run one. This was a cause for concern as the possibility of bias may enter research findings reported by enthusiasts. For example, in enthusiast-dominated research, the placebo effect was not mentioned as a possible explanation for the effects found, although this is common in much mental health research (McGuire 2000). Murray continued that enthusiasm is an important 'ingredient for success' (p. 148), but that it is rarely controlled for.

These two propositions are supported by the suggestion of Deahl and Turner (1997) that few researchers remain in the home treatment services they evaluate: they move on and the demise of the service follows shortly behind them. Conversely, the longevity and continued results of Training in Community Living (Test 1992) and of the Buckingham project (Andrew 1990) would, of course, be examples with which to counter this accusation.

However, with findings that individualised care packages may be dependent on a caregiver's attitudes to management practices (Conning and Rowland 1992), that different processes of care between nurses and social workers often result in the same outcomes for clients (Cawthray et al 1999) and that both individual and service ideologies have differential effects on service delivery (Baker 1982), it can be seen that there is a great need for much more research into the effects of team working on service outcomes. It is conceivable that it may not be staff enthusiasm, but the process of team building and integrated practice in these home treatment teams that results in improved service delivery and thereby accounts for the findings of research in this area.

Further problems and issues

An initial problem when considering research and evaluation of home treatment services is the variety of models in existence – both models of service provision and the evaluation approaches applied to services, as has been seen from the overview of research above. What Hobbs (1984) stated for crisis services can be applied equally to home treatment:

> A variety of techniques are applied in a variety of settings to a wide variety of problems, by practitioners with a variety of skills and qualifications, and with a variety of aims (p. 32).

In the UK most home treatment services set up as an alternative to hospital admission now take on clients for relatively short periods as compared with earlier services which provided both acute and long-term follow-up care.

Uchtenhagen (1986) pointed out that different models of evaluation, including different sources of data, are used to evaluate different types of services. This, in turn, makes it very difficult to draw conclusions about research findings and pinpoint the aspects of service provision or evaluation responsible for the results found. This, coupled with the assertion of Goss and Gluckman (1996) that what works in one area may not do so in another, means that findings from research studies may not be generalisable, as Braun et al (1981) argued, in particular, for home treatment services. An example of this in practice was provided by Test (1992) who found that in adaptations of the psychiatric assertive community treatment model where clients used the services of several mental health providers rather than those of one team, clients showed fewer favourable psychosocial outcomes when compared with the outcomes of the original programme.

One must also consider research in terms of what it purports to measure. Ruggeri and Tansella (1995) made the point that effectiveness (the results of intervention in practice) and efficacy (the potential of an intervention within controlled experimental conditions) are different and that separating experiment from practice is particularly difficult in evaluating psychiatric interventions. Yuen (1994) provided an alternative definition of effectiveness, that of whether clients benefit from the service provided, and distinguished this from the measurement of quality, that is whether service goals are met, but reported that the two were often used interchangeably.

Whether carrying out research or developing services, it is important to start out with definitions of variables that everyone can understand and relate to. It is also important to explicitly identify service and evaluation goals in order for others to see whether these have been addressed. For example, much research claims to show the effectiveness of home treatment and its cost-effectiveness when compared to traditional inpatient services. However, as suggested by Uchtenhagen (1986) the measurement of effectiveness, costs and cost-effectiveness differs widely across studies, as does what is actually reported.

Taking the measurement of costs as a specific example, this has been clearly described by McCrone and Weich (1996), defining direct, indirect and hidden costs. Direct costs accrue through contacts with specialist mental health services. Indirect costs are caused through other health service contacts as a result of mental ill health. Hidden costs are described as the loss of production due to the presence of mental ill health, for example family burden, lost employment or lost leisure time of mental health service users, their families or friends. Unfortunately, much of the research into home treatment services does not adopt this rigour when considering the evaluation of costs. Calculation and the reporting of costs is usually limited to a consideration only of direct costs and any consideration of indirect or hidden costs is not completely enumerated. For example, Burns et al (1993) and Knapp et al (1994) referred to lost employment and family burden without enumerating either.

Hogan and Orme (1999) have suggested that there are further costs, more deeply embedded than those described as hidden by McCrone and Weich (1996), but that with time these can both be identified and quantified. Indeed, it is suggested that only through consideration of all these costs – direct, indirect, hidden and those more deeply embedded (e.g. carer visits to the GP due to experiences of burden, subsequent prescription costs, accidents caused through lack of sleep and so on) – that the full effects of mental ill health and of mental health service interventions may be seen.

It is suggested that the measurement of costs needs to adopt the more thorough approach of cost-benefit analysis described by Weisbrod et al (1980). For example, consideration only of direct costs indicated that the home treatment option of Training in Community Living was 10% more costly than hospital-based treatment. However, when all the costs and benefits were taken together, the home-based option was 5% less expensive than hospital care (Weisbrod et al 1980). In this way any change in the cost burden of different agencies may be accounted for as the cost-benefit analysis approach allows people to see where the changes in the distribution of expenditure have occurred, for example from health to social services.

As with evaluations as a whole, the different approaches taken to measure costs mean that no firm conclusions can be drawn about the overall impact of home treatment services in this area. Services have been found to be cheaper (Fenton et al 1982, Hoult et al 1983, Burns et al 1993, Knapp et al 1994, Minghella et al 1998) and more expensive (Fenton et al 1984) than standard hospital care. It is possible to say that each individual service has had an effect, not that home treatment services *per se*, have a consistent outcome in relation to costs.

Conclusions about cost-effectiveness are also difficult to make. Clear definitions of cost-effectiveness do exist, but are not often reported or considered by researchers. Bowling (1997) defined cost-effectiveness as 'the ratio of the net change in health care costs to the net change in health outcomes' (p. 83). That is, any change in clients' symptoms needs to be related directly to any change in costs. However, the literature suggests this is rarely the case and cost-effectiveness reported for services is often only an indication of cost savings of the home treatment service when compared with a traditional one. One example of an attempt to measure cost-effectiveness as defined would be that of Knapp et al (1994) who linked improvements in client symptomatology to differences in costs of the home treatment and standard care options of the Daily Living Programme in Southwark.

Moving on to consideration of the measurement of client symptomatology, this too is achieved in many different ways, with different researchers and services employing different measures. For example, Stein and Test (1980) utilised the Short Clinical Rating Scale, Hoult et al (1983) used the PSE and BPRS and Minghella et al (1998) used the BPRS and HoNOS. Phelan et al (1995) have commented upon this and others (see Tyrer 1995b) have suggested there is a need to develop a tool that is short enough to be used in routine clinical practice for this purpose. Dean and Foster (1993) pointed out that an alternative measure of the success of treatment programmes would be the extent to which goals set down in individual care plans had been met.

One aspect of services that, to some extent, negates all these approaches to measurement is the ongoing process of change (Uchtenhagen 1986). Services adapt and change rapidly, sometimes as a response to resource limitations or changes in personnel, or in an attempt to improve services for clients. These changes may affect service provision and make any previous evaluation obsolete. For example, introducing a social worker into a nursing service, or extending opening hours to cover the whole 24-hour period, may change the outcomes experienced by clients and a new study will be required to measure the effects of these changes.

Qualitative approaches

The above critique has focused on the more readily quantifiable aspects of research evaluation and highlights problems with this. A more qualitative approach has been adopted by some researchers in the form of the measurement of users' views. The measurement of clients' views of service provision is important as users can report those aspects of care they feel have helped them (Holloway 1993). However, this often becomes a quantitative process too, through the use of questionnaires that ask specific closed questions (Williams 1995).

Client satisfaction has been considered to be indicative of clients' views of services and has been measured in a number of research projects. However, what satisfaction actually means and what satisfaction questionnaires actually measure is debatable. Ricketts (1992) suggested that researchers' ideas of what satisfaction is differ and this results in different ways of measuring satisfaction. Also, the use of questionnaires raises issues that are of interest to researchers or the person who designed the questionnaire and not necessarily to the person responding (Beeforth et al 1990, Williams 1995). Finally, Ruggeri (1996) has suggested that satisfaction questionnaires, particularly those developed in-house, may be inadequate owing to a lack of psychometric properties. That is, some measures may not be sensitive to changes in satisfaction nor actually measure clients' views.

Burns and Santos (1995) reported that any measurement of user satisfaction with home treatment services usually results in a high level of satisfaction being expressed. They suggested that these high rates of satisfaction with home treatment services require further qualitative research in order to understand both why this may be the case and the mechanisms underlying these findings. The simple measuring of client satisfaction therefore needs to move on to a consideration of the specific aspects of care that may account for positive findings regarding home treatment services specifically, and mental health services in general.

Previous research: conclusions

To conclude, although much research has shown individual home treatment services to be effective, to cost less than standard inpatient care, and to be satisfactory to service users, these findings are not generalisable across home treatment services as a whole. The findings of many studies are not comparable as service design and evaluation methods differ greatly. Without explicit definitions and goals of evaluation processes, an amount of critical thinking needs to be employed when reading studies in this area of research, as in all others.

Future research needs

A few suggestions for future research in home treatment have been made in the critique above. For example, the need to look at the underlying causes of client satisfaction and the need for greater use of cost-benefit analysis. Specific questions for future research have also been raised by some. For example, Burns and Santos (1995) suggested further work is required into whether home treatment should be considered:

as an adjunct to other services and treatment, or as a comprehensive and continuous service system for adults with severe mental illness (p. 669).

Considering what has been reported above, it is generally suggested that, in order to aid research and evaluation of services, a clear set of aims and objectives for services is required (Hogan and Orme 1999). Both services and evaluative projects need to explicitly state what it is they intend to achieve for clients and other key stakeholders, in order that it is clear whether or not these goals are met. Goals need to be defined and suitable instruments identified or designed to measure whether or not they are achieved.

The period of time over which evaluations take place and the content of evaluations also need to be borne in mind. Evaluations of home treatment services mainly occur in the short term, and Burns and Santos (1995) suggested this, coupled with the problems of retaining subjects and measuring outcomes, results in inconclusive evidence as to the effects of services. Ruggeri and Tansella (1995) suggested that evaluation is a long-term complex process that needs to consider all levels at which an intervention may be effective. In particular they suggest that studies and services need to consider the patient's view of service effectiveness.

Client satisfaction can be seen to be a nebulous concept (see above) and interviews are to be preferred over the use of questionnaires. Open-ended interviews, although time-consuming, are qualitative and yield information of use – more so than the answers to a set of 'hotel' questions (Williams 1995). Here the user is given time and support to express their feelings about services without feeling pressure to conform to a 'right' set of answers. This process would perhaps benefit from the employment of user-researchers in this interviewing role (Beeforth et al 1990).

Indeed, it is important to ascertain the feelings of all parties involved in home treatment services. Research should focus on the multiple components of care, concentrate on staff, clients and their families, and consider both subjective and objective variables (Ruggeri and Tansella 1995). It is therefore necessary to interview all stakeholders – clients, staff, referrers, service managers and others – in order for them to express their opinions and raise issues of importance to them that may also affect service provision. For example, a GP who has never received any feedback from the local home treatment service may cease to refer clients to it, to the detriment of both the client and the service. Ultimately, all the demonstrations of cost savings and effectiveness are meaningless if the users concerned do not feel that they have benefited in some way from the service.

Returning to specific issues to be addressed by future research, Ruggeri and Tansella (1995) stated that outcomes need to be considered over as wide a range of variables as possible, including quality of life and social support. Coid (1994) suggested that large cohorts of community care clients need to be considered in order to ascertain the relative risks of community-based versus hospital care. Taube et al (1990) described eight improvements to the evaluation of home treatment services, which included:

- comparing home treatment to existing community teams rather than to hospital care
- considering all costs
- trying to distinguish between specific aspects of service provision and outcome
- using longer follow-up periods (at least 18 months).

Additional future needs identified by Tyrer (1995b) relate specifically to staff and include the need to consider turnover in community teams, the occurrence of untoward incidents toward community staff and the effects of community work on staff morale and other elements of staff satisfaction. Specific research in each of these areas is required rather than these issues being considered as part of another piece of work. As has been suggested above, Tyrer added that there is a need to research the constitution of multidisciplinary teams and the qualifications and skills that work best. Also consideration needs to be given to staff training and skills, and how these change or develop through community team working.

Tyrer (1995a) suggested that research needs to identify the negative as well as the positive aspects of home treatment services. Wykes (1995) highlighted the need to research the 'toxicity' of community care in terms of the effects on staff morale, stress, burnout and sickness rates. Again, untoward events, family burden and effects on the wider community need to be considered. Community care failure also requires further research, in order to compare conditions where success and failure occur and to identify those factors that result in the successful implementation of services (Wykes 1995).

Phelan, Strathdee and Thornicroft (1995) described an action plan for researchers that required researchers to support routine evaluation and conduct large-scale randomised controlled trials. They suggested that the effects of services on carers, staff and the wider community need to be investigated and these groups, along with clinicians and users, should be able to guide the direction of research. The dissemination of research findings then needs to be wide – to policy-makers, managers and clinicians – to ensure findings are acted upon.

Tyrer (1995b) included a discussion of the merits and problems of using an RCT approach to research in community care. It was suggested that this approach is suited to comparison of drug effects, but not to the evaluation of therapeutic interventions. However, there is no information from current research as to whether specific interventions may benefit specific populations, and Tyrer suggested this was one area that might benefit from the RCT approach, provided that tighter definitions than previously are employed. Work is also required to see whether or not specific diagnostic groups are more suited to home or hospital treatment.

Regarding the issue of RCTs, the benefits of this approach alone in indicating the efficacy of treatments in mental health have been previously questioned (Task Force on Promotion and Dissemination of Psychological Procedures 1993). Phelan et al (1995) recognised that RCTs may not be feasible in some cases and suggested other forms of controlled research are required, such as observation or survey, to assess the effects of services on clients and the wider community.

Within home treatment programmes it is not possible to place tight controls on the person's whole environment, as in 'laboratory' research. The idea of simulating laboratory conditions in the 'real world' setting is a dubious one (see Ruggeri and Tansella 1995); not only is it dubious ethically, but it promotes a tendency for investigators to think in terms of 'parameters' and 'factors' rather than 'individuals' and 'institutions'. We have already noted the array of independent variables within home treatment that cannot simply be 'controlled' by further strict medical evaluation. 'Strict control' of the study is rarely followed anyway, and many of these projects have been criticised precisely because they are 'pilot' rather than fully 'operational' projects (for example see Thomas et al 1996). At the individual client level, Aptitude X Treatment Interactions (Chambless et al 1996) – individual characteristics such as resistance and degree of socialisation that may affect an individual's response to treatment – are typically unaccounted for and not controlled.

Before-and-after research design programmes assume little or no change during the period of study. This is rarely upheld in practice. For example, Muijen et al (1992) made reference to changes that occurred in the Daily Living Programme in Southwark after a client killed a child. The resulting media coverage led to a lowering of morale in the team and tighter controls on the programme from management. The RCT approach to evaluation does not allow for the investigation of such changes in, and the constraints upon progress of, these studies. For example, any changes in hospital or home treatment staff; the 'Hawthorne effect' created by setting up a new programme and it receiving 'special status' and extra resources (thus, staff morale being abnormally high); changes in policies of the management towards treatments as the research progresses; and changes within the inter-team and inter-agency dynamics (for example see Cohen, Chapter 6, this volume) cannot be accounted for. The fundamental design of the evaluation does not allow adaptation to these possible changes and prevents the researcher from making alterations as a result of changes in circumstances, which frequently arise. The RCT approach may even be detrimental to the programme itself by discouraging new developments and redefinitions midstream.

Imposing artificial and arbitrary restrictions on the scope of a study can be to the detriment of other data, e.g. researcher observations, conversations or other information gleaned from outside the numerical data collection. These forms of data may be discounted as 'subjective', 'anecdotal' or 'impressionistic' despite the possibility of having significant influence for the programme and further explanation of evaluation findings. Research studies using the RCT approach employ large samples and seek statistical generalisations; they therefore tend to be insensitive to atypical results or variations in programmes, despite their significance for innovation or possible importance to the individuals or institutions concerned. Finally, this sort of evaluation often fails to articulate the views of participants, sponsors and other parties who may have stakes in innovative programmes. The idea of seeking objective truths from evaluations often eclipses the need to outline diversity and disparity of the views of different internal groups. For instance, few evaluations of home treatment programmes have sought the views of carers, and fewer have given adequate space to differing views of the project (see Hogan 1997).

Health evaluations performed on projects such as home treatment services will never reach the strict controls required to narrowly compare programmes in a numerical way, and attaining such positivistic research results offers us limited information of the 'real success' (or 'failure') of home treatment programmes. It is understandable that, given time and resource constraints, quantitative monitoring will carry more weight with local management of the schemes in answering the main questions of quality of care, cost-efficiency and diversion from the hospital, but these evaluations often neglect issues of programme development, staff input, dealing with crises and potential problems of the service, and how other services can develop within the community context. Crucially the measures to attain these processes and outcomes need not always be confined to the 'systematic' methods of surveys and questionnaires, but can develop an array of methodologies, which best answer the questions posed by the introduction of a new service and can allow for the acceptance of atypical responses as well as expected ones (Cohen 1999). A move to more qualitative approaches does not have to mean a move to 'woolly' insubstantial research in terms of methods or findings. Stiles (1999) provided a list of criteria for evaluating qualitative research, which applies equally well to quantitative approaches. This list includes stating the questions to be addressed clearly at the outset, providing details on the selection of clients (and an explanation of any changes to this if they happen) and providing details of the methodology of the research such that replication is possible. Additionally, researchers' preconceptions, experiences of the research process and cultural and societal values colour both quantitative and qualitative research and need to be considered by researchers in the development and completion of their work as well as by readers of published findings.

Conclusion

To summarise, this chapter has provided a brief overview of previous research in the area of IHT services and highlighted areas for further development in order to improve both practice and research. Home treatment services have been found to benefit clients and to be valued by them and their carers. The case for the development of these services nationwide within the UK has been made and they are now considered to be a necessary component of routine community-based practice (DoH 1999).

The move to formative rather than summative research is a priority so that evaluations result in service development, rather than 'continuation as normal versus closure' as the only possible outcome. The methodologies to achieve this change in emphasis need to be developed further with a subsequent reduction in the reliance on traditional scientific methods. Finally, with the development of services based on local needs assessment (Minghella et al 1998) and services planned with all involved agencies (DoH 1999), services will be better able meet client, rather than purchaser or provider, need. Generalisation from research findings will therefore become even more difficult. However, as services need to be individualised to meet individual population need, perhaps this can only be a good thing, requiring that services are developed with this in mind and not simply 'copied' from what has gone before.

References

Andrews G (1990) An innovative community psychiatric service. Lancet 335:1087–1088.

Baker F (1982) Effects of value systems on service delivery. In: Schulberg HC, Kililea M, The Modern Practice of Community Mental Health. San Francisco: Jossey-Bass.

Beeforth M, Conlan F, Field V, Hoser B, Sayce L (1990) Whose Service is it Anyway? Users' views on co-ordinating community care. London: Research and Development for Psychiatry.

Bowling A (1997) Research Methods in Health: investigating health and health services. Buckingham: Open University Press.

Braun P, Kochansky G, Shapiro R (1981) Overview: deinstitutionalisation of psychiatric patients, a critical review of outcome studies. American Journal of Psychiatry 138(6):736–749.

Burns BJ, Santos AB (1995) Assertive community treatment: an update of randomized trials. Psychiatric Services 46(7):669–675.

Burns T, Raftery J, Beadsmore A, McGuigan S, Dickson M (1993) A controlled trial of home-based active psychiatric services II: treatment patterns and costs. British Journal of Psychiatry 163:55–61.

Burti L, Tansella M (1995) Acute home-based care and community psychiatry. In: Phelan M, Strathdee G, Thornicroft G, Emergency Mental Health Services in the Community. Cambridge: Cambridge University Press.

Cawthray S, Whelen E, Wells S (1999) An Evaluation of Crisis Services for the Mentally Ill in Wirral. Report for Wirral Health Authority.

Chambless DL, Sanderson WC, Shoham V et al (1996) An update on empirically validated therapies. Clinical Psychologist 49:5–18.

Coates DB et al (1976) Evaluating hospital and home treatment for psychiatric patients. Canada's Mental Health 24:28–33.

Cohen BMZ (1999) Psychiatric User Narratives. Bradford: University of Bradford.

Coid J (1994) Failure in community care: psychiatry's dilemma. British Medical Journal 308:805–806.

Conning AM, Rowland LA (1992) Staff attitudes and the provision of individualised care: what determines what we do for people with long-term psychiatric disabilities? Journal of Mental Health 1:71–80.

Deahl M, Turner T (1997) General psychiatry in no-man's land. British Journal of Psychiatry 171:6–8.

Dean C, Foster A (1993) Measuring outcomes. In: Dean C, Freeman H, Community Mental Health Care. International perspectives on making it happen. London: Gaskell.

Dean C, Phillips J, Gadd M, Joseph M, England S (1993) Comparison of community based service with hospital based service for people with acute, severe psychiatric illness. British Medical Journal 307:473–476.

Dedman P (1993) Home treatment for acute psychiatric disorder. British Medical Journal 306:1359–1360.

DoH (1999) A National Service Framework for Mental Health. London: HMSO.

Fenton FR et al (1979) A comparative trial of home and hospital psychiatric care. Archives of General Psychiatry 36:1073–1079.

Fenton FR, Tessier L, Contandriopoulos A-P, Nguyen H, Struening EL (1982) A comparative trial of home and hospital psychiatric treatment: financial costs. Canadian Journal of Psychiatry 27(3):177–187.

Fenton FR, Tessier L, Struening EL et al (1984) A two-year follow-up of a comparative trial of cost-effectiveness of home and hospital psychiatric treatment. Canadian Journal of Psychiatry 29(3):205–211.

Godfrey M, Townsend J (1995) Intensive home treatment team: users' and carers' experiences of the service and the outcome of care (Working Paper 1). Leeds: Nuffield Institute for Health/University of Leeds.

Goss T, Gluckman P (1996) Developing a mental health focus for purchasers. In: Thornicroft G, Strathdee G, Commissioning Mental Health Services. London: HMSO.

Hobbs M (1984) Crisis intervention in theory in practice: a selective review. British Journal of Medical Psychology 57:23–34.

Hogan K (1997) The effectiveness of crisis service: a review of research. Paper presented at the 2nd Annual Conference on Crisis Services in Mental Health, University of Leeds.

Hogan K, Crawford-Wright A, Orme S, Easthope Y, Baker D (1997) Walsall Crisis Support Service Final Report, Volume 2: Literature review. Wolverhampton: University of Wolverhampton.

Hogan K, Orme S (1999) The effectiveness of crisis services. In: Tomlinson D, Allen K, Crisis Services and Hospital Crises: Mental Health at a Turning Point. Aldershot: Ashgate.

Holloway F (1993) The user perspective on mental health services: its value and limitations. In: Leiper R, Field V, Counting for Something in Mental Health Service: Effective user feedback. Aldershot: Avebury.

Hoult J, Reynolds I, Charbonneau-Powis M, Weekes P, Briggs J (1983) Psychiatric hospital versus community treatment: the results of a randomised trial. Australian and New Zealand Journal of Psychiatry 17:160–167.

Kiesler K (1982) Mental hospital and alternative care: noninstitutionalisation as potential public policy for mental patients. American Psychologist 37(4):349–360.

Knapp M, Beecham J, Koutsogeorgopoulou V et al (1994) Service use and cost of home-based versus hospital-based care for people with serious mental illness. British Journal of Psychiatry 165:195–203.

McCrone P, Weich S (1996) Mental health care costs: paucity of measurement. In: Thornicroft G, Tansella M, Mental Health Outcome Measures. Berlin: Springer-Verlag.

McGuire PA (2000) New hope for people with schizophrenia. Monitor on Psychology 31(2).

Minghella E, Ford R, Freeman T, Hoult J, McGlynn P (1998) Open All Hours. London: Sainsbury Centre for Mental Health.

Muijen M et al (1992) Home based care and standard hospital care for patients with severe mental illness: a randomised controlled trial. British Medical Journal 304:749–754.

Pai S, Kapur RL (1983) Evaluation of home care treatment for schizophrenic patients. Acta Psychiatrica Scandinavica 67:80–88.

Phelan M, Strathdee G, Thornicroft G (1995) The future of mental health emergency services. In: Phelan M, Strathdee G, Thornicroft G, Emergency Mental Health Services in the Community. Cambridge: Cambridge University Press.

Pigott HE, Trott L (1993) Translating research into practice: the implementation of an in-home crisis intervention triage and treatment service in the private sector. American College of Medical Quality 8(3):138–144.

Querido A (1968) The shaping of community mental health care. British Journal of Psychiatry 114:293–302.

Ricketts T (1992) Consumer satisfaction surveys in mental health. British Journal of Nursing 1:523–527.

Ruggeri M (1996) Satisfaction with psychiatric services. In: Thornicroft G, Tansella M, Mental Health Outcome Measures. Berlin: Springer-Verlag.

Ruggeri M, Tansella M (1995) Evaluating outcome in mental health care. Current Opinion in Psychiatry 8:116–121.

Sashidharan SP, Smyth M (1992) Evaluation of Home Treatment in Ladywood: results from the first two years. Birmingham: Birmingham Home Treatment Service.

Stein LI, Test MA (1980) Alternative to mental hospital treatment: I. Conceptual model, treatment program, and clinical expectation. Archives of General Psychiatry 37:392–397.

Stein LI, Test MA, Marx AJ (1975) Alternative to the hospital: a controlled study. American Journal of Psychiatry 132(5):517–522.

Stiles WB (1999) Evaluating qualitative research. Evidence-Based Mental Health 2(4):99–101.

Task Force on Promotion and Dissemination of Psychological Procedures (1993) Report adopted by the Division 12 Board – October 1993. American Psychological Association.

Taube CA, Morlock L, Burns BA, Santos AB (1990) New directions in research on assertive community treatment. Hospital and Community Psychiatry 41(6):642–647.

Test MA (1992) Training in Community Living. In: Liberman RP, Handbook of Psychiatric Rehabilitation. London: Macmillan.

Test MA, Stein LI (1980) Alternatives to mental hospital treatment: III Social costs. Archives of General Psychiatry 37:409–412.

Thomas P, Greenwood M, Kearney G, Murray I (1996) The first twelve months of a community support bed unit. Psychiatric Bulletin 20:455–458.

Tyrer P (1995a) Essential issues in community psychiatry. In: Tyrer P, Creed F, Community Psychiatry in Action. Analysis and prospects. Cambridge: Cambridge University Press.

Tyrer P (1995b) Future research strategies. In: Tyrer P, Creed F, Community Psychiatry in Action. Analysis and prospects. Cambridge: Cambridge University Press.

Uchtenhagen A (1986) Evaluation of Community Services. Acta Psychiatrica Belgica 86:350–361.

Weisbrod BA, Test MA, Stein LI (1980) Alternatives to mental hospital treatment: II – Economic benefit–cost analysis. Archives of General Psychiatry 37:400–405.

Whittle P, Mitchell S (1997) Community alternatives project: an evaluation of a community-based acute psychiatric team providing alternatives to admission. Journal of Mental Health 6(4):417–427.

Williams B (1995) Users' views of community mental health care. In: Crosby C, Barry MM, Community Care: Evaluation of the provision of mental health services. Aldershot: Avebury.

Wykes T (1995) The toxicity of community care. In: Tyrer P, Creed F, Community Psychiatry in Action. Analysis and prospects. Cambridge: Cambridge University Press.

Yuen F (1994) Evaluations in mental health services: some methodological considerations. Journal of Nursing Management 2:287–291.

CHAPTER 4

Assessment in crisis/ home treatment services

NEIL BRIMBLECOMBE

Summary

The increase in the number of home treatment services offering crisis assessments is described. Those aspects of assessment particularly important in crisis/home treatment assessments are discussed, with the importance of filtering referrals and gathering information in advance being highlighted. A framework for decision-making is provided.

In the UK there has been a recent rise in the number of services offering intensive home treatment (IHT) as an alternative to psychiatric inpatient admission (see Orme, Chapter 2, this volume). In the past the majority of crisis assessments have been carried out in Accident and Emergency departments or psychiatric units (often by junior psychiatrists alone) or through domiciliary visits by consultants at the request of GPs. Although there have been a number of crisis intervention teams working on the principle of providing rapid response multidisciplinary assessments for psychiatric (or occasionally psychosocial) emergencies for many years, these have not been widely spread (Faulkner et al 1994) and may be handicapped by an inability to offer the intensive follow-up required to provide treatment to those with acute mental health problems severe enough to otherwise warrant admission.

The emphasis within the National Service Framework for Mental Health (DoH 1999) on the need to provide easily accessible 24-hour emergency assessments will lead to further expansion of numbers of emergency assessment services, frequently linked to home treatment teams.

Currently there are two typical structures for assessing for home treatment as an alternative to hospital admission.

- Some home treatment services act as a crisis assessment service in their own right, seeing the majority of urgent referrals or those potentially requiring hospital admission in their catchment area.
- Others take referrals predominantly from other psychiatric services, where an initial crisis assessment has, effectively, already been carried out, for example by a duty doctor in an Accident and Emergency department. The home treatment service then does a follow-up assessment to check that home treatment is actually viable and desirable as an alternative to admission.

Although many aspects of psychiatric assessment remain the same in whatever environment they are carried out, this chapter will focus on those features of assessment which are particularly important in an emergency community assessment. These features are summarised as: pre-assessment issues, the assessment, the decision-making process and the plan of care.

Pre-assessment issues

Filtering and referral criteria

All crisis and IHT services require explicit referral criteria and a process of filtering out those that fail to meet those criteria. Eligibility criteria should be as clear as possible in order to ensure that clients seen are those for whom the service was actually designed. Kwakwa (1995) illustrates the importance of this point in describing a rapid assessment and home treatment service in Cornwall. The client group had changed from that originally targeted, i.e. the severely mentally ill requiring admission, to a group who would previously not have received substantial levels of service input. Furthermore, so much time was spent in carrying out 'rapid assessments' that little was left for actually providing IHT.

Screening serves as an initial assessment (Tufnell et al 1988), increasing the efficiency of services and reducing the likelihood of inappropriate use. Other professionals may be keen to pass on their anxieties about their own clients to emergency services (Drake and Brimblecombe 1999) and evidence exists that such services often receive 'inappropriate' referrals (De La Cour and Dorey 1997). A description of the impact of initial screening was provided by the North Islington Urgent Assessment Service (Crawford et al 1996), where 29% ($n = 42$) of referrals were not seen as suitable for assessment, either because they lived outside the catchment area or because their problems were not considered to need an urgent response.

The screening function is a skilled one, requiring good clinical knowledge and an ability to focus on those most salient points of presentation, particularly in assisting the referrer to identify elements of risk if they exist. Considerable interpersonal communication skills are also required, and assertiveness when the referrer's perception of need is not the same as the screening worker's. A sound knowledge of other local services is also a prerequisite, so that referrers can be redirected to more appropriate agencies rather than merely being refused a service.

Typical reasons for referral are likely to be similar to those found with the Psychiatric Emergency Team in North Birmingham (Minghella et al 1998): onset or relapse of psychotic symptoms, and risk of harm to self or others. Other reasons may include: other symptoms (e.g. panic), not taking medication, and the client's family seeking admission. These problems demand a wide range of skills for any assessors, including:

- risk assessment knowledge and skills
- knowledge of psychological, pharmacological and social interventions with psychosis
- the ability to assess and work with families.

Beyond specific clinical skills and knowledge, assessors require the ability to:

- communicate clearly with others
- act with common sense
- remain calm in a crisis.

In addition to taking the main reason for referral and historical information, the worker must also ascertain whether the client and family are aware of the referral. If other family members are not aware of the referral then consideration should be given to a possible breach of confidentiality simply by an assessing team arriving on the doorstep.

There are very few occasions on which a client should not be told in advance of referral, not only because of common politeness, but also on the practical grounds that arriving unannounced is unlikely to facilitate the forming of a trusting relationship. Exceptions may be made in serious cases where the client might otherwise avoid the assessment, and this might be harmful in terms of risk to self or others, or lead to other undesirable occurrences, such as being picked up by the police.

Once the worker taking the referral is clear that the client's problems appear to meet the service's criteria for assessment, a decision must be taken about the speed of response. Most emergency services have a minimum response time: 2–4 hours is common, a day at the most. The worker needs to balance how urgent the needs of the referred client are with organisational constraints and the needs of other clients. Someone threatening imminent suicide may well need to be seen within 2 hours, someone with a 3-month history of self-neglect may not.

Information gathering

There is an argument that entering an assessment with a mind clear of preconceptions or previous knowledge of the client will allow for more balanced assessment, untainted by labelling. However, this possible advantage is markedly outweighed by that gained through gathering as much information as possible about the client before the assessment. Information can be retrieved both from written records and from those who know the referred individual (Brown 1998). There may be value in contacting both mental health professionals and others, e.g. GPs, social workers, health visitors, etc.

Investigating in advance may save time in the longer term. Where good information exists this may provide direct benefit in removing the need to go over basic background information at the assessment, which may be repetitive to the client and time-consuming to the assessors. There may be important information about side effects of medication recorded previously, which the clients themselves may not be in a position to give accurate information on.

Historical information may be of particular value in beginning to assess the possibility of risk to others (including the assessors), with previous violence being the best predictor of future violence. A history of sexual abuse may suggest a particular need to consider the gender composition of the assessing team. Information about the language spoken or any specific cultural issues should lead to careful consideration as to who needs to be present, for example an interpreter or, preferably, a staff member who can speak the same tongue and/or is sensitive to particular cultural issues.

All previously recorded information is potentially useful, but it should be treated with an open mind. For example, diagnostic labels such as 'personality disorder' may more accurately reflect negative feelings of professionals towards an individual than an objective diagnosis (Lewis and Appleby 1988). Ideally the assessing team should be entering the assessment well informed, but without prejudging the problem or outcome.

Staff safety

As already mentioned, the information gathering process must include enquiries about current or past violence. Resentment or aggression can often be detected by speaking to the referred individual by phone before face-to-face assessment. Decisions need to be made as to how the assessment can be made acceptably risk free for staff. Consideration needs to be given to who should be present, including gender mix, and in the most extreme cases whether the police should attend. Different venues provide different levels of security. Although there are distinct advantages to home assessments (see below) they may also be the most potentially dangerous, with a lack of others to call on in an emergency. An assessment at a community mental health centre or a GP's surgery may decrease risk, although careful consideration should be given as to whether this is simply transferring risk to others, e.g. reception staff.

More generally, the whereabouts of staff should always be recorded and procedures should be in place for following up the late return of members of staff. Mobile phones have some value, mostly as a form of reassurance. Staff training is another key issue in increasing safety. This needs to include general understanding about factors increasing and decreasing aggression, interpersonal skills and physical techniques to allow escape from physical assault. Undoubtedly the environment in which teams operate should influence procedures, with inner city teams having different levels of concern from those operating in rural areas. For example, all visits by the central Manchester Home Option Service after 5 p.m. are carried out in pairs.

When starting an assessment, care should be taken to ensure that exits from the room are not obstructed, so that staff members can leave rapidly should this be necessary. It is also vital that the client is able to leave easily; any perception of being trapped may increase an aggressive response.

The assessing team

The constitution of the assessing team potentially influences the outcome of the assessment as well as the form it may take. There are undoubtedly advantages in assessment by more than one discipline. This allows for the utilisation of a wider range of skills, as well as providing an additional benefit in improving safety (Sutherby and Szmukler 1995).

In providing assessment to individuals with an acute mental health problem severe enough to potentially warrant admission, in the majority of cases there is a need for a psychiatrist to participate. Medication is likely to play a role in any subsequent home treatment, either in terms of treating an underlying condition or in alleviating distressing symptoms such as sleeplessness. A medical opinion may also be of particular value in considering the possible role of any physical factors.

The presence of other disciplines at an assessment, e.g. nursing or social work, is equally important, providing different perspectives. Burns et al (1993) describe a community service, which although with no more resources than other services, significantly reduced the number of hospital admissions. The authors speculated that this may have been largely due to the active participation of non-medical disciplines in the assessment process, as opposed to other services where initial assessments were carried out by psychiatrists and other disciplines became involved at a later point. For any home treatment service it is also vital that someone participates in the assessment who is aware of all the practical day-to-day issues involved in providing IHT. This person would commonly, but not invariably, be a nurse.

Additional to the assessment team from the home treatment service, it is often valuable to have other involved professionals present, e.g. community mental health team key workers. This assists in ensuring continuity of care (Coleman et al 1998) and helps the home treatment/crisis team assessors in providing insights from someone who knows the client and their normal presentation. The presence of a worker familiar to the client may also be of value in reducing any anxiety the client may feel in meeting 'strangers' and may be more likely to encourage openness. There may be more general advantages as well in working closely with workers from other services, encouraging good communication and transparent decision making.

However, there is also a need to balance the advantages of having a number of staff present at assessment, with all the various contributions they can each bring, with the danger of having too many people there, which can be extremely intimidating or provocative to the client. This situation may be aggravated by the commitment most health and social care workers have to training others in their professions. The guiding rule needs always to be that the presence of students/trainees should not be detrimental to the client's sense of well-being and whenever possible should be agreed in advance.

Although those attending the assessment are responsible for the process of assessment itself, there is often value in having others available to discuss particularly difficult issues that may arise. A system of on-call senior staff may provide direct advice or, more frequently, simply a fresh view of a situation. Emergency assessment services obviously have to act quickly, but it is very rare that a situation is such that a few minutes cannot be taken to step out of the assessment situation either to discuss issues among the assessing team or to telephone someone else for advice or discussion.

Carers and others

Apart from the professionals involved in the assessment the client may wish to arrange to have someone else present at the interview, either as moral support or to help clarify points that the client does not feel able to do themselves. Such individuals may also help to understand any cultural issues that the assessor may not be aware of.

Family members may provide useful additional information which may be of particular value if the client tends to minimise the seriousness of their problems, or simply has no insight into having a problem at all. Noting any strain on, or distress of, relatives is an important feature of an emergency community assessment and of the decision-making process (see below). There is a risk, however, that the client will become alienated if the assessors are seen as 'taking the side' of relatives. Whenever possible all contacts with relatives should be agreed with the client and the client should be given the opportunity to be seen alone, without the relatives present. If a family member is also involved in the referral, there may be benefit in seeking collateral information from other family members, especially if there is evidence of conflict or markedly differing views between client and the referring family member.

Issues at assessment

The setting

There are distinct advantages to be gained from carrying out assessments in the client's own home. The client can be seen functioning in their normal environment. Clients often feel more secure and better understood in their own homes. Jones et al (1987) found that 80% of clients seen by a multidisciplinary team for community-based assessments felt that the workers had understood their difficulties better by seeing them in their own homes. Many clients will prefer to be seen in their own home rather than a 'stigmatising' psychiatric facility, with continued negative media attention to the mentally ill (Philo 1998). However, visiting a home address may have similar effects; numbers of mental health workers arriving armed with briefcases may cause equal distress through drawing the attention of neighbours.

Much can be gained from viewing the home itself, its condition often saying much about the condition of the client. Self-neglect may be demonstrated through the state of hygiene and organisation, although, as in all aspects of assessment, the norms of the client rather than those of the assessors should provide the key frame of reference. More generally, aspects of personality can be suggested through furnishings and belongings which may not be gathered in a normal psychiatric interview. Cases of hoarding are an extreme example. Bizarre decor, such as silver foil on walls, will rapidly suggest areas for further enquiry with the client. Where there is concern about levels of self-care, food supplies can be checked with the client's permission. Risk, especially to the elderly or physically weak, can be considered through noting the adequacy of heating or risks from ill-placed fires. The security of a home can be evaluated where there is risk of exploitation from others.

Another potential benefit might arise simply from having an assessment away from a psychiatric facility, as some authors have noted an increased likelihood of admission when assessments take place at a 'hospital' (Friedman et al 1964, Dean and Gadd 1990). There may be an expectation created in the mind of both client and any carer that an admission will inevitably take place once a hospital's doors are crossed, and this may be exacerbated when a considerable distance has been travelled to reach the institution. Sometimes, of course, the place of assessment may simply reflect a higher level of disturbance in the client, e.g. if an individual is brought to hospital under Section 136 of the Mental Health Act.

The assessment

The initial period of any assessment is crucial to establishing an environment which allows for the detail of assessment to take place. Assessors should take care as to the pace at which they proceed, showing sensitivity to the presentation and concerns of the client. Commonly held fears of clients may include:

- being taken to hospital against their will
- social services removing their children
- not being listened to (often based on previous negative experiences)
- being labelled 'mad'.

Adopting a friendly but professional manner and giving some brief information about the service is often useful to begin an exchange of information. Giving time for the client or carer to ask questions initially may allow them to dispel misconceptions or fears early on.

Although the initial aim is always to carry out a full assessment at the initial meeting, in some cases this will not be possible. The client may find talking difficult or may not be able to concentrate for a long enough period, or may simply be unwilling to discuss certain issues at that time. In such cases an assessment may need to be continued over two or more meetings. This is, of course, dependent on the absence of indicators which suggest immediate risk.

History from the client

A useful point to begin is to establish with the client why they believe the assessment is taking place. This begins to establish their view about their own problems. When a carer or other professional has made the referral, the client's understanding of this may also throw considerable light on the dynamics involved in that relationship. Where the problem exists in the minds of someone other than the client, this begins to suggest that any intervention required may need to be with that person instead of, or as well as with, the client themselves.

The use of active listening skills encourages the client to express thoughts and feelings. Restating the client's words back to them demonstrates that they are being listened to and ensures that the assessors actually do understand what is being said to them.

Mental state examination

A detailed description of this process is beyond the remit of this chapter, but attempts must always be made to adequately assess each of the following components.

- The interview should make note of the client's appearance and behaviour, including the nature of the contact established between the assessing team and the client.
- Aspects of speech, including its spontaneity, rate and volume, as well as any particular preoccupations which surface, provide useful ways of trying to understand the client's state of mind.
- Mood can be explored through both direct questions and through noting the client's view of their circumstances. Biological features of mood disturbance can be identified through ascertaining whether there are changes in the areas of sleep, appetite, libido and energy levels.

- Thought disorder is often revealed through the general process of interviewing, but direct questions may be needed to ascertain whether the client is experiencing hallucinations in any form.
- Any disorientation in time, person or place and any obvious lapses in memory will indicate the need for further investigation.

Coping mechanisms

Crisis theory sees the genesis of a crisis arising through the inability of an individual's usual coping mechanisms to deal with a novel problem (Caplan 1964). Although crisis theory may not always be readily applicable in working with individuals with severe mental health problems (see Chapter 1), ascertaining how difficulties are typically dealt with, both individually and within a family, provides useful information, especially as attempted solutions may easily become part of the problem (Weakland et al 1974); for example, 'having a little drink to help me relax'. Alternatively, a client's usually positive ways of coping may be being underused for a variety of reasons, and part of a treatment plan may be helping the client to build on existing strengths.

Social environment

A significant difference in emphasis between a 'standard' psychiatric assessment and that carried out by a home treatment/crisis service is the need for a wider assessment of the functioning of the individual in their social context (Sutherby and Szmukler 1995). The need for detailed social information may often be neglected in an inpatient setting where the client's temporary separation from their usual environment and the adoption of the role of the inpatient can provide a false dichotomy between psychopathology and environment. Social factors will inevitably affect the mental state of the client for either good or ill, regardless of the presence of any serious mental health problem. Campbell and Szmukler (1993) provide a useful framework with which to assess the social resources of a client. This includes detailed consideration of: accommodation, finances, home activities, outside activities and information concerning carers, formal and informal.

This information helps inform the decision as to the viability of home treatment and, if this is the outcome, will then provide information on which an initial care plan can be based, with any problems (and strengths) having been identified.

Cultural factors

Definitions of 'normality' vary markedly between different cultures (Helman 1990), and there are always risks involved in largely middle-class British mental health professionals making judgements as to the 'appropriateness' of behaviour in those from other cultures. Stress and distress are also likely to be experienced and presented in different ways, such as in the degree of somatisation expressed (Mumford 1995).

The assessing team cannot be expected to be well informed about the nuances of every cultural tradition, but should be aware to apply value judgements cautiously and seek more informed help where there is doubt. Beyond this, the assessment of individuals from minorities must be considered in the broader social context. Assessors may potentially be seen as representative of repressive or racist authority. Paranoia or uncooperativeness that may be detected on assessment may, when based on bad past experiences, be a reasonable response on the client's behalf rather than a sign of psychopathology (Littlewood and Lipsedge 1982).

A number of home treatment services have striven to ensure that their staff reflect the ethnic mix in the areas they serve, providing both cultural awareness and an ability to relate to clients in their first language without the interpersonal clumsiness afforded by the use of professional interpreters or the undesirable use of family or friends as informal, but not objective, interpreters.

Child care

Although direct assessment of the well-being of any child in the household is beyond the remit of an emergency psychiatric assessment service, the observable interaction between child and client may suggest difficulties in this area. Clearly any evidence of neglect or mistreatment requires further investigation, and if there is evidence of risk to a child social services will need to be informed. When this is the case, wherever possible the client should be encouraged to be involved in this process. When there is no such evidence, but it is clear that the client is in need of practical assistance in the short term because of their mental state, then the assessors can offer to be intermediaries with other services or offer advice about availability of such services.

Financial status

The finances of an individual may be important to an assessment in a number of ways. Financial strains, through debts or simply due to inadequate income, constitute a very common stressor. Questions can be asked about income and outgoings and whether help has been obtained, for example through contacting social security offices or gaining advice from the Citizens' Advice Bureau. A second common problem may arise through overspending due to a mental health problem. Questions about recent expenditure may demonstrate disinhibition where this is a change from previous patterns.

Daily living skills

Vital skills involved in maintenance of physical and social well-being include shopping, cooking and paying bills. In terms of influencing decision-making about the most appropriate form of intervention it is useful to try and separate out any recent changes, i.e. deterioration in skills arising from a psychiatric illness or psychosocial crisis, from longer-term issues relating to an enduring mental health problem or simple lack of skills.

Physical examination

An estimated 33.5–80% of 'psychiatric patients' suffer from physical illnesses requiring treatment, with about half of these conditions being unrecognised (Hall et al 1981). Home treatment assessors need to be aware that concomitant physical problems may worsen or even cause psychological or behavioural problems. For example, a close relationship has been identified between the onset of depression and physical ill health (Prince et al 1998).

A convincing argument can be put forward for the need for physical examinations to be carried out at the commencement of home treatment, as practised in some areas currently (e.g. the Bradford Home Treatment Service). Certainly blood investigations should be routinely carried out by teams' medical staff. Specific physical investigations may be required before the commencement of some treatments, e.g. lithium therapy and electroconvulsive therapy (ECT). More generally, any specific issues of concern may require close liaison with the client's GP.

Substance misuse

Enquiry must be made into the presence and level of any drug and alcohol use. This has implications in terms of both treatment and treatability. Persistent heavy use of alcohol or illicit drugs can make interventions in the community very difficult and potentially danger-ous if prescription medication is provided as well.

Where there is a possibility that illicit drugs may have played a part in causing the current disturbance, then drug screens can occa-sionally be a useful tool when the client is willing to agree to this.

The decision-making process

A key issue for any emergency service is that of admission – when is it really necessary? There is evidence of marked differences between areas (and individual clinicians) as to what constitutes an adequate reason for admission in general psychiatry (Flannigan et al 1984). A complicated interplay of several factors is likely to influence assessors in their attempts to decide whether home treatment is a suitable alternative to admission in each individual case. A division can be made between those factors statistically linked with an increased likelihood of admission and the actual process whereby decisions are made.

Predicting outcomes

Any service offering IHT will inevitably admit a proportion of those assessed. Currently there exists little research as to which character-istics of assessed individuals are likely to be related to an increased likelihood that home treatment can be offered rather than admis-sion. A study in North Birmingham of the Psychiatric Emergency Team (Minghella et al 1998) showed an initial admission rate of 34% ($n = 20$) of a total sample of 58, and three more clients were admitted after 'minimal' intervention from the team.

In central Manchester, Harrison et al (1999) found that those admitted to an inpatient unit, rather than being provided with home treatment, were seen as being more likely to present with 'attention-seeking behaviour', bizarre speech content, incoherent speech, socially unacceptable habits and overactivity. Clients treated by the home treatment service were seen as presenting more frequently with suicidal ideation or with eating and drinking problems. Generally, those requiring inpatient care were seen as presenting with disturbed behaviour or aggression.

Diagnosis has been claimed to be related to an increased likelihood of admission as opposed to home treatment, for example with individuals with personality disorders (Tufnell et al 1988, Brimblecombe and O'Sullivan 1999, Bracken and Cohen 1999). This may relate to both impulsiveness and the difficulties with which such individuals often have in negotiating in a meaningful way. However, significant numbers of individuals with such a diagnosis still appear to be successfully treated at home.

Home treatment or hospital?

Pioneers of home treatment Marx, Test and Stein (1973) suggested that hospital be reserved for patients who are so

> severely and acutely psychotic or depressed as to require imminent somatic therapy only feasible in the hospital's high structure environment and necessitating good nursing care.

More recently, Harrison et al (1999) have suggested a framework of factors which are key to deciding whether home treatment is a viable and desirable option to admission, through: 'identification of risk, compliance with the service, support networks and home circumstances'.

Tufnell et al (1988) provide a similar framework for decision-making concerning the ability of a service to contain the immediate crisis at home. The variables include:

- risk involved in any home treatment being manageable
- willingness of the client to accept home treatment
- enough support being available and willingly given by family and/or neighbours
- lack of need for specific hospital-based treatments
- the availability and adequacy of other community services.

Having established the viability of home treatment, the next stage is to establish whether home treatment is not only viable, but also desirable (Sutherby and Szmukler 1995).

Risk

Shergill and Szmukler (1998) point out that although many community mental health clients are at a theoretical risk of harming themselves or others, such acts are actually statistically quite rare. The difficulties of prediction of such low frequency events is 'intractable', yet mental health professionals need to address this issue in the interests of their clients, others and themselves, to demonstrate they have acted professionally.

The frequency with which risk to self is quoted as the main reason for admission can be very high (Brimblecombe and O'Sullivan 1999), which illustrates the importance of such risk in decision-making about home treatment vs. admission. Some features associated with increased risk to self are listed in Table 4.1.

Table 4.1: Selected features increasing risk to self

Male gender	Elderly males
Young adult males	Young Asian females
Previous attempts	Physical illness
Living alone	Access to means of suicide
Bereavement in childhood	Social class I and V
Not employed	Previous aggressive behaviour
Recent contact with GP	Recent discharge from ward
Threats of self-harm	Recent clinical improvement

Although the presence of suicidal ideation does increase the likelihood of admission, the majority of such individuals can be treated at home (Brimblecombe 2000). The key issue is likely to be the ability of the client to state that they will not harm themselves before the next visit or will contact the team should they feel they are no longer able to control an impulse to self-harm. Such an agreement will only be acceptable where the assessors believe that the client, firstly, is being honest about this, and, secondly, has the capacity to show such control. Clearly much rests on the assessors' subjective view of these factors, which will be based largely on 'gut feeling', where there is no previous history to base such decisions on. In some cases the client agreeing to the removal of means of self-harm, such as medication or car keys, may be important both practically and symbolically.

Admissions due to risk to others constitute a small, but significant, proportion of total admissions where home treatment is otherwise available (Brimblecombe and O'Sullivan 1999). Part of any assessment of risk to others needs to include a specific evaluation of possible risks to home treatment staff. Where there is some risk, but considered manageable in a setting other than the client's home, then a key feature influencing decision-making as to the viability of avoiding hospital admission may be the client's willingness to attend a local office rather than be seen at home. Some features consistent with increased risk to others are listed in Table 4.2.

Table 4.2: Selected features increasing risk to others

History of violence	Sustained anger or fear
History of threats	Plans for, and fantasies of, attack
Persecutory delusions with fear of imminent attack	Escalating conflict with specific individuals
Morbid jealousy	Impulsivity
Involvement of close relative or companion in conflict arising from delusional convictions	Substance abuse
Clouding of consciousness and confusion	

Compliance with the service

Issues concerning compliance can take a number of forms. All home treatment services have found a significant minority of clients who simply prefer to be treated in hospital, despite being offered the alternative of home treatment, which makes the possibility of home treatment very problematic. This group of clients can constitute as much as a quarter of all admissions at the point of initial assessment (Brimblecombe and O'Sullivan 1999). However, most studies show the majority of those who have received both home-based and hospital-based treatment prefer the home option. For example, Cohen (1999) found that, in Bradford, of 52 clients who had received home treatment and had also previously been in hospital, 81% thought home treatment to be in some way better than hospital, with just 12% thinking the opposite. Those preferring hospital treatment commented on their wish to escape troubles and the outside world, and to be looked after. The availability of food, accommodation, financial help, 24-hour care, company and activities were all mentioned.

A second form of non-compliance is that the client simply does not agree with the treatment plan, despite attempts to negotiate this. This is normally linked to the client's non-acceptance of the necessity for any treatment. Such numbers are likely to be relatively small (Brimblecombe and O'Sullivan 1999) and often lead onto a Mental Health Act assessment, dependent on the severity of the problem.

Support by family

The roles, attitudes and availability of family and carers is often a significant issue at assessment. Early home treatment services required all those offered acute community-based care as an alternative to hospital admission to be living with families (Langsley et al 1968) or having family members willing to assist in treatment (Fenton, Tessier and Struening 1979), but subsequently this was found not to be an absolute prerequisite. However, living alone may still be related to an increase in the likelihood of admission at initial assessment (Dean and Gadd 1990). This may arise partially from the characteristics of some individuals who live alone, e.g. poorer social skills, greater isolation and, partially, from the greatly enhanced opportunities someone living with a carer may have in terms of increased supervision and support.

In an Australian study of individuals presenting to a home treatment service for the first time with psychotic illness, Fitzgerald and Kulkarni (1998) found that where raters scored levels of family support low at initial assessment, then there subsequently proved to be an increased chance of home treatment not being successful. Beyond this, the work of Vaughan and Leff (1976) illustrates that high levels of negative expressed emotion within a family can be positively harmful to those diagnosed with schizophrenia, increasing the risk of relapse. Such negative family dynamics may not necessarily lead to admission, as educating the family can become part of the community-based care of the client (Francell, Conn and Gray 1988).

Conversely, the needs of family and carer must be considered, as the burden associated with home treatment should not be unacceptable for them, even with the high levels of support that are available from such services. There is no evidence that most carers prefer admission where an alternative of IHT is available (Marks et al 1994), although there is a need for home treatment services to take into account that supporting carers in their caring role may not be enough, and that they have needs in their own right which might also need to be addressed (Godfrey 1996). It may be particularly important to explain clearly to carers about the availability of easily accessible support from a home treatment service, as well as the relative frequency of visits available. This is especially so where the only experience carers have had in previous crises is that there is an unpalatable choice between low levels of support from generic community services or relief through hospital admission.

More generally there is a need to consider the needs of the individual with the general principle of community care that

> the demands which different groups of ill or disabled people make in total upon the community must not be greater than the community can accept. (HMSO 1975)

This is not to advocate bowing to prejudice by removing anyone acting in an 'abnormal' way from the community, but acknowledges that where behaviour causes genuine distress to others, then professionals have a duty to take this into consideration.

Need for hospital-based treatments

There are few hard and fast rules about when a treatment is required which can only be provided in a hospital setting, when intensive levels of observation are required in clients presenting at high risk. Alcohol detoxification may need to take place in hospital where there is a history of serious withdrawals or no carer is present to alert services in the event of physical complications. There may be a need to commence an individual on medication in hospital where there is a licensing requirement that requires this.

For other treatments individual circumstances are all-important. Electroconvulsive therapy (ECT), for example, may often be provided on an outpatient basis, especially with the aid of an IHT team. However, this may be considered too risky if the client is in a weak physical condition or there is evidence that any sudden increase in energy levels in a depressed and retarded client may unacceptably increase the risk of suicide. Similarly, where a high level of physical care is required in terms of ensuring adequate diet and hygiene this may often be provided at home when very frequent visits and a clear and detailed care plan can ensure that an individual's needs are met. Contextual factors may mitigate against this option, for example if the client is physically very weak or access may be difficult.

Where very high levels of tranquillising antipsychotic medication are required (even in the absence of other serious risk) this may need to take place in hospital owing to the need for very close monitoring for unwanted effects. However, this again depends on a range of factors, such as dosages, previous response and the presence of carers to alert about side effects.

There are other things available in hospital that may not be found in the community, although they could only loosely be described as 'treatment'. There are specific psychological connotations of being in a hospital environment, such as the feeling of containment and being 'cared for'. Where individuals feel particularly 'out of control' or overwhelmingly emotionally needy, for some the only way these needs can be met is in a very structured environment with staff present 24 hours a day (Godfrey 1996, Cohen 1999). This is the exception, and even where it is required it should only be provided for short periods of time, else the solution to the problem becomes part of the problem through fostering a dependency on the institution.

Other community services

An IHT service may be able to supply high levels of input in terms of home visits offering treatment, support and monitoring, but in many cases the availability of other resources plays an important role in making home care feasible. A common example is day care. This is especially valuable where an individual is isolated and reintegration with others is a key aspect to the care plan. Day care can also be of particular value in providing respite for carers or family, or alternatively providing respite for the client from their family. The availability of a meals-on-wheels service may ensure the availability of a hot meal once a day, in addition to food that can be prepared with the help of home treatment staff. In some areas the availability of short-term alternative accommodation has allowed clients to remain out of hospital where otherwise the home situation would not allow this (Turkington, Kingdon and Malcolm 1991, Whittle and Mitchell 1997).

Desirability

A series of issues will influence views on the desirability of home treatment, as opposed to just its viability. Anyone working within a home treatment or crisis service is likely to hold the general view that clients have the right to be treated in the least restrictive environment possible. They may also hold that, generally, coping skills and autonomy are best learnt in the community (Stein, Test and Marx 1975). However, there is a need to consider each client's needs on an individual basis. Having established that home treatment for an individual is viable, the next question will therefore need to exclude the possibility that hospital admission may be the more therapeutic option: 'what will admittance to hospital provide that cannot be provided through intensive home care?' (Smyth and Bracken 1994). In some cases the answer to this will be suggested by past history, for example, if the client had previously not responded well to home treatment, but had done well in hospital.

The plan of care

Where the decision is taken to offer IHT as an alternative to admission, the final stage of an assessment must involve negotiating the details of the plan of care between the assessors and client, involving carers where appropriate. The assessors may propose a plan and listen to whether it is acceptable in its proposed form or whether reasonable requests are made to make changes. A willingness to negotiate is essential, although clearly if the client declines to accept so much of a care plan that the benefits of treatment are negated or that the risk involved would be unacceptably high, then the decision to offer home treatment will inevitably require reconsideration.

Having agreed what the care is for and broadly how it will be delivered, information should be given (preferably in written form) about how to contact the home treatment service in emergencies.

Following on from the agreement of a general plan of care, the assessing team must ensure that one individual is nominated as key worker for the client, to ensure that a more detailed care plan is established and that care is properly coordinated. Another immediate post-assessment task is to ensure that information concerning the outcome is passed on to both the referrer and to other services involved with the client.

Once home treatment begins, the need for assessment is not over. Part of home treatment must be continuous reassessment, both in terms of identifying changing needs and, most importantly, in terms of changing risk. The most common reason for hospital admission once home treatment has begun is increase in risk, either to others or to self (Minghella et al 1998, Brimblecombe and O'Sullivan 1999).

References

Bracken P, Cohen B (1999) Home treatment in Bradford. Psychiatric Bulletin 23:349–352.

Brimblecombe N (2000) Suicidal ideation, home treatment and admission. Mental Health Nursing 20(1):22–26.

Brimblecombe N, O'Sullivan G (1999) Diagnosis, assessments and admissions from a community treatment team. Psychiatric Bulletin 23:72–74.

Brown T (1998) Psychiatric emergencies. Advances in Psychiatric Treatment 4:270–276.

Burns T, Beadsmore A, Bhat AV, Oliver A, Mathers C (1993) A controlled trial of home-based acute psychiatric services. I: Clinical and social outcome. British Journal of Psychiatry 163:49–54.

Campbell PG, Szmukler GI (1993) The Social State: a proposed new element in the standard psychiatric assessment. Psychiatric Bulletin 17:4–7.

Caplan G (1964) Principles of Preventive Psychiatry. London: Tavistock.

Cohen BMZ (1999) Innovatory forms of evaluation for new crisis services. Science, Discourse and Mind 1(1):12–31.

Coleman M, Donnelly P, Davies A, Brace P (1998) Evaluating intensive support in community mental health care. Mental Health Nursing 18(5):8–11.

Crawford MJ, Kohen D, Dalton J (1996) Evaluation of a community based service for urgent psychiatric assessment. Psychiatric Bulletin 20:592–595.

De La Cour J, Dorey T (1997) The need for a CPN rapid response service. Mental Health Nursing 17:18–21.

Dean C, Gadd EM (1990) Home treatment for acute psychiatric illness. British Medical Journal 301:1021–1023.

DoH (1999) National Service Framework for Mental Health. Modern Standards and Service Models. London: Department of Health.

Drake M, Brimblecombe N (1999) Stress in mental health nursing: comparing teams. Mental Health Nursing 19(1):14–19.

Faulkner A, Field V, Muijen M (1994) A Survey of Adult Mental Health Services. London: Sainsbury Centre.

Fenton FR, Tessier L, Struening EL (1979) A comparative trial of home and hospital psychiatric care. Archives of General Psychiatry 36:1073–1079.

Fitzgerald P, Kulkarni J (1998) Home-oriented management programme for people with early psychosis. British Journal of Psychiatry 172(suppl 33):39–44.

Flannigan C, Glover G, Wing J, Lewis S, Bebbington P, Feeney S (1984) Inner London collaborative audit of admission in two health districts. III: Reasons for acute admission to psychiatric wards. British Journal of Psychiatry 165:750–759.

Francell CG, Conn VS, Gray DP (1988) Families' perceptions of burden of care for chronic mentally ill relatives. Hospital and Community Psychiatry 39(12):1296–1300.

Friedman TT, Becker A, Weiner L (1964) The psychiatric home treatment service: preliminary report of five years of clinical experience. American Journal of Psychiatry 120:782–788.

Godfrey M (1996) User and carer outcomes in mental health. Outcome briefings. Nuffield Institute for Health 8:17–20.

Hall RC, Warrdner ER, Popkin MK et al (1981) Unrecognised physical illness prompting psychiatric admission: a prospective study. American Journal of Psychiatry 138:629–635.

Harrison J, Poynton A, Marshall J, Gater R, Creed F (1999) Open all hours: extending the role of the psychiatric day hospital. Psychiatric Bulletin 23:400–404.

HMSO (1975) Better Services for the Mentally Ill. Cmnd 6223. London: HMSO.

Helman CG (1990) Culture, Health and Illness, 2nd edn. Oxford: Butterworth-Heinemann.

Jones SJ, Turner RJ, Grant JE (1987) Assessing patients in their homes. Bulletin of the Royal College of Psychiatry 11:117–119.

Kwakwa J (1995) Alternatives to hospital-based mental health care. Nursing Times 91(23):38–39.

Langsley DG, Pittman FS, Machotka P, Flomenhaft K (1968) Family crisis therapy – results and implications. Family Process 7(2):145–158.

Lewis G, Appleby L (1988) Personality disorder: the patients psychiatrists dislike. British Journal of Psychiatry 153:44–49.

Littlewood R, Lipsedge M (1982) Aliens and Alienists. Ethnic minorities and psychiatry. Harmondsworth: Penguin.

Marks IM, Connolly J, Muijen M, Audini B, McNamee G, Lawrence RE (1994) Home-based versus hospital-based care for people with serious mental illness. British Journal of Psychiatry 165:179–194.

Marx AJ, Test MA, Stein LI (1973) Extrahospital management of severe mental illness. Archives of General Psychiatry 29:205–511.

Minghella E, Ford R, Freeman T, Hoult J, McGlynn P, O'Halloran P (1998) Open All Hours. 24-hour response for people with mental health emergencies. London: Sainsbury Centre for Mental Health.

Mumford DB (1995) Cultural issues in assessment and treatment. Current Opinion in Psychiatry 8:134–137.

Philo G (1998) The media and mental health promotion. Mental Health Review 3(2):21–25.

Prince MJ, Harwood RH, Thomas A et al (1998) A prospective population-based cohort study of the effects of disablement and social milieu on the onset and maintenance of late-life depression. The Gospel Oak Project VII. Psychological Medicine 28:337–350.

Shergill SS, Szmukler G (1998) How predictable is violence and suicide in community psychiatric practice? Journal of Mental Health 7(4):393–401.

Smyth M, Bracken P (1994) Senior registrar training in home treatment. Psychiatric Bulletin 18:408–409.

Stein LI, Test MA, Marx AJ (1975) Alternative to the hospital: a controlled study. American Journal of Psychiatry 132(5):517–522.

Sutherby K, Szmukler G (1995) Community assessment of crisis. In: Phelan M, Strathdee G, Thornicroft G (eds) Emergency Mental Health Services in the Community. Cambridge: Cambridge University Press.

Tufnell G, Bouras N, Watson JP, Brough DI (1988) Home assessment and treatment in a community psychiatric service. Acta Psychiatrica Scandinavica 72:20–28.

Turkington D, Kingdon D, Malcolm K (1991) The use of an unstaffed flat for crisis intervention and rehabilitation. Psychiatric Bulletin 15:13–14.

Vaughan C, Leff J (1976) The influence of family and social factors on the course of psychiatric illness: a comparison of schizophrenic and depressed neurotic patients. British Journal of Psychiatry 129:125–137.

Weakland JH, Fisch R, Watzlawick P, Bodin AM (1974) Brief therapy: focused problem resolution. Family Process 13(2):141–168.

Whittle P, Mitchell S (1997) Community alternatives project: An evaluation of a community-based acute psychiatric team providing alternatives to admission. Journal of Mental Health 6(4):417–427.

CHAPTER 5

'With a slightly lighter heart . . . '
Mental Health Act Assessments: Does a home treatment team make a difference?

Louise M. Dunn

Summary

Research into the application of the Mental Health Act is summarised. A comparison is made between Mental Health Act assessments in two areas, one with an acute home treatment team and one without. The views of professionals involved in assessments are explored and conclusions drawn.

When it comes to the care and treatment of those suffering from mental distress, each age has had its particular approach, based largely on prevailing contemporary philosophies and what they have had to say about human nature, the human condition, society, 'sanity' and 'dangerousness' (Foucault 1967, Bean and Mounser 1993). The 'big idea' of the second half of the twentieth century was that large-scale incarceration was no longer desirable or justifiable as a response to a problem seen variously as spiritual, moral, philosophical, economic and, finally, medical. The developing climate of civil rights, individual freedom and self-determination permeated the field of psychiatry, giving voice to disquiet about the process by which people could be detained and treated against their will. One response to this was the announcement in 1961 by Enoch Powell, Minister of Health, that care in the community was to be the new policy, thus shifting the focus of care away from large institutions.

The development of services consistent with this policy has been slow and uneven, but there has been an interest among mental health professionals for some time in the possibility and effectiveness of home treatment for acute mental distress. The history, successes and otherwise of this idea are described elsewhere in this book.

Another major development was the passing of the Mental Health Act in 1983. Concern about medical dominance, along with an acknowledgement of the developing emphasis on social factors and civil rights, were reflected in the new legislation. An important innovation was the creation of the approved social worker (ASW); he or she is involved alongside doctors in deciding whether admission to hospital is necessary, even against the wishes of the client. The ASW's duties include those of considering the social context of the client, seeking alternatives to admission and ensuring that the outcome is the least restrictive possible in the circumstances.

Viable alternatives need to be available to the ASW in order that these duties can be carried out meaningfully, and it is here that the Mental Health Act meets home treatment. Where it exists, it should represent an opportunity, under certain circumstances, to avoid detention by providing just such an alternative.

The project described here which was supported by the Institute of Psychiatry and Southwark Social Services, sought to investigate whether the existence of a service, which was designed to offer a direct alternative to hospital admission, had any effect on the numbers and circumstances of Mental Health Act assessments in its area, during the year of study. A comparison was made with an area which was largely similar, but which did not have this service.

Previous research

The research relevant to this project is dominated by two large studies into the activities of ASWs, and their implementation of the 1983 Mental Health Act.

The earliest and largest was that carried out by Barnes, Bowl and Fisher (1990), which examined Mental Health Act assessments shortly after the implementation of the legislation. It investigated some 7000 assessments between 1985 and 1986 among a population of 16 million people, in local authorities all over the country. The second study was by Hatfield, Mohamad and Huxley (1992) and was explicitly similar in design and method to that by Barnes et al (1990). It was smaller in scale, though still extensive, and investigated 1262 assessments between 1989 and 1990, among a population of 1 million people.

These studies were particularly interested in, and critical of, the extent to which ASWs were seen to have embraced their responsibility to look at the client's social context, to provide a balance to the medical view and to look for possible alternatives to admission. They acknowledge a lack of alternatives on which ASWs could draw, and there are suggestions that more crisis facilities should have been available. Many of the alternatives suggested by the authors, such as social work support or recourse to GP input, seem more applicable to continuing care rather than to the crisis situations most often faced in a Mental Health Act assessment.

Home treatment studies

In comparison with the Mental Health Act, home treatment benefits from a large body of research, which is discussed in more detail elsewhere in this book. Randomised trials of hospital versus community treatment, dating from 1967 (Pasamanick et al 1967) and continuing up to the present day, consistently concluded that home treatment gave outcomes on clinical and social measures which were at least equal to hospital care. Examples come from Britain (Dean et al 1993, Marks et al 1994), Australia (Hoult, Rosen and Reynolds 1984), the US (Stein and Test 1980) and Canada (Fenton, Tessier and Struening 1979). Difficulties in generalising results may occur, because the studies involved are based on different models, with, for example, varying conditions to which the control populations are subject. There were also differences in inclusion criteria, and in the nature and quality of the services which form the point of comparison. These may have represented 'standard hospital care' (Simpson, Seager and Robertson 1993), for example, which may have been of indifferent quality, or at least not comparable with modern well-developed community mental health services.

Holloway (1995) asserts that there seems to be some 'misunderstanding' of the early work on home treatment; although patients in all of the studies were accepted as acutely ill, the length of the experiments and the methods adopted relate more to longer-term, on-going, rather than acute, care. The Daily Living Programme, for example, offered social and problem-solving interventions over a period of at least 20 months (Marks et al 1994). This combination of acute care and longer-term medical and social care seems to reflect the service offered by the whole range of mental health services in the areas of the present study.

In conclusion, the fact is that the ASW studies discussed here took place before the general development of home treatment schemes, and so were not able to evaluate this alternative form of care and its effect on matters surrounding formal assessments in any detail. There has been very little research linking the two areas, which is the object of the project described here.

As home treatment becomes more widely available, one might expect it to have effects on assessments in a number of ways: it could reduce the numbers of assessments and affect the type of people undergoing them, or the decisions made. This study was designed to explore these areas by using record data to compare the numbers, circumstances and outcomes of formal assessments undertaken in two areas, one with a home treatment service and one without (Dunn 2001).

The research

In England and Wales, when a person is suffering from a mental disorder serious enough to indicate a possible need for hospitalisation, perhaps against their wishes, this may give rise to a request for a formal assessment to be undertaken under the terms of the Mental Health Act 1983. This requires an ASW and (usually) two doctors, one of whom must be qualified in psychiatry, to interview the client and make a decision based on as much information and understanding of the whole situation as possible.

The areas

The aim of this study was to compare the circumstances and outcomes of Mental Health Act assessments undertaken in two areas of a particular county. The areas were broadly similar in a number of respects such as service provision, policy and social demography, but differed in that one of the areas had the services of a team whose aim is to provide rapid response and home treatment for people in acute psychiatric distress, as an alternative to admission. The object was to examine whether there were any differences that might be associated with this extra service.

One of the areas was to the north of the county, and the other to the west; they are therefore called North and West in this chapter. Each comprised a new town and included a smaller, older town and outlying villages. The populations of North and West (for those aged over 16) are 89 584 and 105 134 respectively. Thus they differed in size, but a number of indicators showed that they had much in common. On a socio-demographic level, their social class/employment profiles were comparable. They have similar rankings on the Jarman Index (North 2582, West 2669; HCC 1996), with North being very slightly more deprived socially.

To measure the relative mental health needs of the areas, the Mental Illness Needs Index (MINI) computer program (Glover et al 1995) was consulted and it was found that the areas appeared to have similar levels of need: see Figure 5.1. As can be seen, North comes out as very slightly more needy, but, one would argue, not enough to invalidate the assertion that the areas are comparable.

Both areas were served by multidisciplinary community mental health teams (CMHTs), in which specialist social workers and community psychiatric nurses (CPNs) worked together with consultant

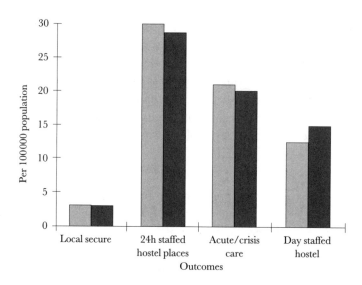

Figure 5.1: A comparison of estimated mental health needs, in terms of places required per 100 000 population. Four selected types of resource. Light bars, North; dark bars, West.

psychiatrists and junior doctors. North had access to the well-established psychiatric wings of two large local general hospitals and a large area hospital which specialised in caring for people with severe mental illness of organic origin. West's services included two new psychiatric units, which had replaced a large traditional asylum in the previous 2 years. Services were older and more established in North; in West the CMHT was finally established as a joint team in 1993.

In terms of services, North workers had a number of services available, which included:

- access to home care staff, who specialised in providing domiciliary care to people with mental health problems
- a day hospital operating 5 days a week
- the use of the hospital ward at weekends for day care
- night sitters.

An important contribution was made by the non-medical support team run by the local social services, which could operate 7 days a week, and could offer practical and social support at home for people whose needs were mainly long term. Offering social care, this team was not comparable with the home treatment team, which formed part of the study described below. This team in North was different from the home treatment team in West in that it was non-medical in approach and in the training and qualifications of its staff. West had the services of a support team run by the health service, originally set up to offer intensive home support to long-term patients discharged to their own (new) homes when the hospital closed down. It offered long-term medical and social care, caring for about 14 clients, and had later accepted other people with long-term psychiatric problems. It had one 'crisis bed', which could be used for 24-hour emergency care for its own or other clients. During the period of study there was no day hospital available for West, though there was day care for non-crisis situations. Both areas shared the services of countywide hostels, which were not able to offer a crisis response.

Approved social workers (ASWs) in both areas worked for the same county council social services department and thus were subject to the same policies, refresher training and management.

The community treatment team (CTT)

The explicit purpose of this service was to offer prompt assessment, and home treatment, as an alternative to admission to people who 'may be suffering from an acute mental health problem serious enough to warrant admission' (WHCH 1997). It operated 7 days a week between the hours of 9 a.m. and 11 p.m. and comprised nine qualified CPNs, one part-time consultant and one staff-grade psychiatrist.

It excluded people under 16 years old, those with organic disorder and those in the care of the health-run support team, as well as those with a primary substance abuse problem, except where the recently established home detoxification service was offered. It also worked with people to effect early discharge from hospital.

Design

This was a record-based comparative study which monitored the circumstances and outcomes of Mental Health Act assessments in two areas over a 1-year period, from the beginning of March 1996 until the end of February 1997. This time period was chosen because it produced sufficient data to lend itself to meaningful analysis, and was long enough to cover all seasons and to account for busy and quiet periods. It covered the same length of time as Barnes, Bowl and Fisher (1990) and Hatfield, Mohamad and Huxley (1992), which were used as a point of reference. March 1996 was also the time from which the CTT was able to offer a fully staffed service that included full medical cover.

Data were extracted from reports written by ASWs after each assessment, in which they are required to give details of the circumstances, decision-making and outcome of the assessment to show that legal requirements have been met. As a result, it was necessary to rely on information routinely recorded in the reports, and so it was not possible to collect data about matters such as class or employment circumstances, or details about the quality of family relationships. It is true that this method of extracting information had limitations, in that, for example, triangulation of methods was not applied. Resources did not allow for this, but it is also true that the reports used were very detailed and written to a high standard, as required by the policy of the social services responsible.

The sample included all Mental Health Act assessments in the study period, of individuals with home addresses in the two areas. People from other areas and of no fixed abode were excluded, as they would not have been eligible for CTT intervention.

With respect to 'diagnosis', information derived from the reports was sometimes implicit, but usually explicit. It was not necessarily the result of tight operational definitions.

Results

After excluding eight assessments from the total carried out during the year in question because they lived outside the county or were of no fixed abode, 181 remained to be analysed. These related to 129 individual people; of these, 22 were assessed twice, 10 three times, 2 four times and 1 person underwent five assessments. The remainder (94) were assessed just once. The data collected in the project were analysed in two ways, in relation to incidents and to individuals, as appropriate.

The hypothesis was that the CTT could influence assessments in a number of ways: it could reduce their numbers by absorbing people becoming unwell before the need for a crisis assessment, or it could have some effect on the timing of an assessment in an illness episode, perhaps making it happen later rather than earlier. It could affect the profile of people being referred for assessment. The balance and nature of outcomes might be affected because of the nature of the CTT as an explicit alternative to admission.

The simplest way of looking at this, initially, was to compare relative rates of assessments for the populations as a whole. The populations of North and West differ in size, but were comparable in various socio-demographic details, as described above. Numbers of assessments for the year under review, after the exclusions noted above, are: 95 in North and 86 in West.

The rates of Mental Health Act assessments, per 100 000 adult population, were 107 for North and 81 for West (Herts Social Services 1997). Thus rates of assessments were considerably lower in the larger district, by the order of about 25%. This proportional and absolute difference indicated that further investigation was warranted.

There was a significant difference in type of outcome between areas ($\chi^2 = 9.54$, $df = 4$, $p = < 0.046$). Detentions under Section 3 of the Mental Health Act were more likely to occur in North, where such decisions comprised 41.3% of all outcomes. In West, Section 3 decisions comprised 31.7% of the total; although this is lower, it places this area in line with the average for the county, which was 32.9% for Section 3 decisions (Herts Social Services 1997). See Figure 5.2.

Evidence of any possible filtering effect of the CTT can be looked for in differences in the characteristics of people presenting in the two areas. It may be that different sorts of people reach the point of a formal assessment in each area, given the different community services. There is some evidence of their impact to be found in the CTT's own figures relating to their overall activity. For example, most (88%) of their work derived from referrals of people in the community believed by the referrer to be suffering from a mental health problem acute enough for hospital admission (WHCH 1997). With a 'take on' rate of 51% (of some 400 referrals per year) it is reasonable to assume a degree of filtering of people who might otherwise, without access to crisis services, have reached a point at which a Mental Health Act assessment was necessary.

In order to explore whether differing filtering processes were in operation, an analysis of a range of variables was undertaken. Comparisons of results in the two areas relating to many personal characteristics were made, and did not show any significant statistical

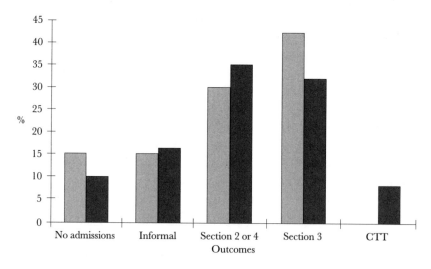

Figure 5.2: Outcome of assessments by area. Light bars, North; dark bars, West.

differences ($p > 0.05$). These included: living circumstances; ethnic origin; gender; a substance abuse problem; the presence of a learning disability or other organic diagnosis; age and diagnosis by gender. With respect to the assessment process itself, there were, again, no significant differences. These included: police involvement; the participation of doctors known to the client; legal status before the assessment; the issue of violence: and knowledge of the client by the service.

Though results fell short of statistical significance, one of the most interesting findings to emerge related to the re-referral during the year in question of a number of people. This seemed to account to a very large extent for the higher number of assessments in North. West had a higher proportion of first, and a lower proportion of subsequent, assessments (see Table 5.1).

Table 5.1: A comparison of the numbers of re-referrals by area

	North	West	Total
	% (n)	% (n)	n
First assessment	66.3 (63)	76.7 (66)	129
Subsequent assessment	33.7 (32)	23.3 (20)	52
Total	100.0 (95)	100.0 (86)	181

Examining the gender breakdown, it can be seen that males referred more than once seemed to account for the greater numbers in North (see Table 5.2).

Table 5.2: Inter-area comparison of men re-referred for assessment within the year of study

	North	West	Total
	% (n)	% (n)	n
First assessment	63.2 (36)	81.8 (36)	72
Subsequent assessment	36.8 (21)	18.2 (8)	29
Total	100.0 (57)	100.0 (44)	101

$\chi^2 = 4.22$, $df = 1$, $p = < 0.039$

Exploring further, it was found that with respect to diagnosis of re-referred individuals, 17 in North and 12 in West were diagnosed as having a 'psychosis'. Some of this finding is possibly explained by the fact that the sample included several young people who seemed to be undergoing the early emergence of a psychotic illness, during which it is often not possible to make a definitive diagnosis and start a full treatment plan. It also confirms a finding by Turner, Ness and Imison (1992) that multiple presentation and psychotic illness are often associated. Examination of CTT records might throw some light on the question of whether they have nevertheless been able to absorb proportionally more people in this group. With respect to the personality disorder category, one individual accounted for five of the total of ten assessments in that group in West, with another cropping up three times.

CTT records show that 56.4% of their referrals were of people already receiving a mental health service (WHCH 1997). This enables one to hypothesise that this team was the factor which effectively reduced the number of potential repeated referrals for assessment under the Mental Health Act, a point which will be developed below.

The effects of home treatment in West

When gauging the effectiveness of the CTT it is important to be clear about the nature of their potential 'clientele'. This was done by removing from the calculations all the people excluded by their criteria, such as all those with a known diagnosis of mental health problems organic in origin, those under the care of the home support team, and those with a primary diagnosis of learning disability.

The result was to leave a total of 63 assessments of people potentially eligible to be cared for by the CTT. Looking at the numbers of assessments during which the CTT were recorded as having been consulted, or borne in mind by the ASW, and when they were available as an option (i.e. not in the middle of the night), the total was 35 out of 79 assessments (44.3%). They were used as an alternative to hospital admission on 17.3% of the occasions on which they were consulted (see Figure 5.3).

The most marked difference in outcome between those who had CTT input into their assessment and those who did not was the likelihood of being detained under Section 3, the treatment section, which is for people who are already known. In fact it appears that a

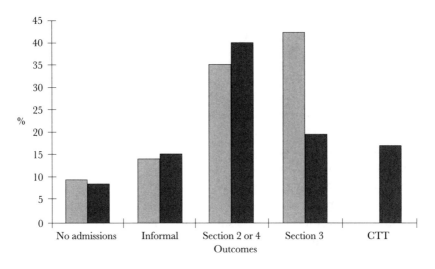

Figure 5.3: Outcome of assessments in the presence (dark bars) or absence (light bars) of CTT consultation.

Section 3 is some 46% more likely if the CTT is not considered as an option. It may be that where the CTT was not consulted, it was already known to the assessors that the person was not suitable for home treatment, owing to violence, to previous failed attempts, or perhaps to an unacceptable risk of self-harm. Further analysis revealed that of all those detained under Section 3, about a quarter were being seen by the CTT before the assessment, indicating that home treatment had been tried. Analysis of the perceived risks indicated that danger to the self was the most common reason given for admission, which ties in with the CTT's own figures for those admitted from their care (WHCH 1997).

To summarise, an analysis of the data indicated that differences between the areas could be traced to three related factors. Firstly, broadly speaking, numbers in West were lower for all diagnostic and socio-demographic groups. However, the rate of re-referrals seemed to provide the most likely explanation for the higher numbers in North – 32 to West's 20. Investigation revealed that the largest recurring group in both areas was that of people diagnosed as 'psychotic', which replicated a finding by Hatfield, Mohamad and Huxley (1992) that an increasing number of assessments nationally is largely accounted for by repeated referrals of young men with diagnoses of schizophrenia.

A second discovery was that of a smaller likelihood of a Section 3 decision as an outcome in West, though the statistics do not reach significance, and mirror overall county figures. In addition, within West, the fact of having had the CTT involved in an assessment again decreased the likelihood of Section 3 being the outcome by a much larger amount, in the order of about 46%. The issues of the 'revolving door' and treatment (Section 3) orders seem to be connected here, in that they relate to known people. If one adds a third factor, that of the home treatment service performing a filtering function, in that it can take early referral of and quick action with people who are already known, it can be argued that this could account for lower levels of assessments in its area. Potential Section 3 candidates may have been absorbed and dealt with before a crisis point was reached, or in a way more acceptable to someone reluctant to go to hospital. Thus this effect of the CTT was seen in inter-area comparisons, as well as within the area, when assessments involving, or not involving, the CTT were compared.

Conclusions should be considered with the context of the study in mind. The CTT exists and was established alongside relatively well-developed community mental health services in both areas. Acute intervention can be followed up by other elements of the service, replicating in some ways the regime tried by the Daily Living Programme (Marks et al 1994), and in West the health-run longer-term support team can provide the whole range of response for a limited number of people.

The view from the ground

The study included in-depth semi-structured interviews with a dozen staff members, such as consultant psychiatrists, registrars, senior house officers and ASWs, whose work involves them routinely with the carrying out of Mental Health Act assessments. Their views were sought about a range of issues surrounding assessments, and particularly about alternatives to admission or detention in hospital, as well as the impact of a home treatment service on these matters.

Interestingly, staff in the area which does not have a home treatment service did not mention it as an option when asked to suggest desirable alternatives, a finding which is not exclusive to this study (Flannigan et al 1984, Fulop et al 1996). Virtually all the ASWs questioned spoke about 'crisis houses' or 'crash pads' as being desirable alternative disposals for someone in acute mental distress. These were not closely defined, but seemed to allude to places which, if they existed, could allow people to 'be mentally ill', to have time out, to be free to work through their crises while being supported, without the stigma of psychiatric hospital admission. It may be that this concept represents a – perhaps fading – echo of ideas popular in psychiatry in the 1960s. Mental illness, or, more specifically, psychosis, was seen by some observers both outside and within psychiatry as perhaps an inner journey of discovery, available to particular people, from which they returned 'to the normal world, . . . with insights different from those of the inhabitants who never embarked on such a voyage' (Bateson in Showalter 1987). There certainly seems, implicit in this idea, the confidence that such a crisis could well resolve itself without medical intervention. The only example of such a solution was one situation described by an ASW which she had resolved, some years before, by the use of a residential establishment run on purely psychodynamic lines. If such facilities, of safe, non-medical crisis support, were available, one ASW pointed out that it could allow for the constructive use of the 14 days available to the ASW following the completion of medical recommendations, thus making the assessment less hurried.

Day hospitals were mentioned as resources which could provide safety, respite for carers, nursing care and – vitally, perhaps – the necessary dimension of 'containment' or 'holding' (Bion in Grotstein 1981) which is often relevant for people in acute distress. Adequately qualified night sitters or even home carers were suggested as resources which might allow patients to remain safely at home, and more help with life crises was felt to be a possible way of reducing the need for admission further down the line. One of the doctors spoke about Community Treatment Orders as a development which could increase the likelihood of someone being able to avoid compulsory admission to hospital. Whether the client would see this as a meaningful alternative, however, is open to debate.

Some of the ideas expressed about possible alternatives were in effect improvements to the home treatment service as it exists. For example, some respondents suggested that a service providing 24-hour care, or at least longer periods of attendance than the CTT are able to give, would be preferable. This tied in with the perception expressed by one worker that the acceptance of clients by the CTT was in part dependent on their readiness to accept medication, helping to impart an image of the CTT being heavily reliant on the 'medical model'. A couple of respondents thought that the CTT were not able to commit the time and resources which would be involved in working with clients who are difficult to engage and who could benefit from lengthy and patient attention, with the object of building trust and reaching a non-crisis resolution.

Two respondents suggested that the CTT had no bearing on the threshold for detention under the Mental Health Act, but might have an effect on that for informal admission. A doctor expressed the view that home treatment and formal assessments were not associated, because a person willing to accept home treatment would therefore not be able to be detained under the terms of the Act. However, others thought that many clients, even in crisis, might resist admission to hospital, but accept treatment at home. This would perhaps be more likely to be the case in situations where administering treatment was the main issue, rather than risk or dangerousness.

When considering whom the service might benefit, professionals' ideas agreed largely with the eligibility criteria of the CTT itself. Home treatment was thought to be suitable in cases of severe but not life-threatening depression, or where members of the client's family or other support networks at home could cope with professional assistance. The self-neglecting elderly were thought to be possible candidates, although people suffering from dementia are excluded from CTT criteria. More than one person considered that the important factor was severity of the mental distress, rather than the type, or diagnosis. The fact that the service could provide for a relatively safe period of assessment, in situations where the extent or exact nature of the problem was unclear, was regarded very positively. This might also allow for the use of the 14-day breathing space mentioned above.

It was considered by most respondents that people for whom home treatment was not a viable alternative to detention included those whose suicidal ideas or feelings put them at serious risk, who had a lack of support at home, or whose carers were unable or unwilling to continue to cope. Clients who needed nursing care for lengthy continuous periods, and throughout the night, were not thought to be suitable candidates because the service as it exists in the area cannot cater for this need. Those who were 'highly aroused', who were unpredictable or uncooperative, and perhaps psychotic, were also considered to be unlikely beneficiaries. Some respondents added to this list people with severe personality disorders or a tendency towards violence.

All of the workers interviewed saw the home treatment service as a 'huge plus', which helped the assessing team to carry out a better assessment. The majority of respondents acknowledged the contribution of the team to the assessment process as a 'very real alternative in many cases'. It was felt to enhance the assessment process, in that it provided the sort of alternative which made the duty of the ASW in this area much more meaningful. Thus the assessment was seen to be broader, 'more thorough', and therefore 'more respectful', in the context of the county being described by one respondent as 'a wilderness' with respect to alternatives. One member of the social services out-of-hours team, whose work covers the whole county, thought that the home treatment service offered an 'excellent alternative' to admission. The worker made the point that the CTT could make an impact by being present at the assessment, thus providing for a realistic appraisal of whether home treatment could be an option. The worker's experience was, however, that the CTT were more often involved in having tried to treat the client at home before the calling of the statutory assessment, signalling that this disposal was not viable. Their contribution lay, therefore, in providing evidence for the ASW and the assessing team of attempts to avoid admission, as well as information about the situation, contributing to a more thorough assessment. This worker made the point that the CTT were easy to contact when needed, in contrast to services in other parts of the county, which could be used but were less readily reachable. Finally, the comment was made that the CTT have sometimes offered to assess and to take on a client for whom the out-of-hours team was arranging an assessment, a move which was often unexpected and pleasing.

It is perhaps important at this juncture to put these views in perspective. The CTT were used as an alternative to hospital on 17% of the occasions on which they were consulted. This figure is not easily interpreted, because, for example, some of the clients involved will have already been cared for or assessed by the CTT and deemed not, or no longer, suitable for home treatment. However, what is notable is the fact that they were consulted in less than half the cases where people eligible for their service were to be assessed. The CTT wish to be involved in all appropriate assessments, and good practice would support this, but the figures were not as encouraging as they could have been.

In looking at the impact of the CTT on Mental Health Act assessments, the study concentrated on a small aspect of the overall phenomenon of home treatment as it exists in the area concerned. The team's work is much broader, and is concerned with providing alternatives to admission in as many cases as possible, as well as the facilitation of early discharge from hospital and support during periods of leave. When discussing the issues with respondents, the matter of statutory assessments sometimes tended to merge with that of admission generally, as people discussed how far the team could provide a service designed to prevent or to delay admission to hospital. Of course, one might suggest that these issues are connected, in that the service makes possible a continuum of care which is more comprehensive, and of which the statutory assessment represents the final stage.

Two clients

To illustrate this point, and to give a human face to the discussion, it might be useful to give one or two examples of the work of the CTT.

One client who has been helped on many occasions is Mrs J, a woman in her 60s who suffers from bipolar affective disorder. She is seen regularly by her key worker, a member of the local Community Mental Health Team, who provides emotional and practical support, and who monitors her mental health. She has had a number of mental health crises over the last few years, during which she typically becomes extremely agitated, has persecutory ideas and sleeps very little. The CTT has normally responded by visiting Mrs J every day, sometimes more than once, to oversee medication, to offer reassurance, to support her carer and to monitor risk. Hospital admission has been unavoidable on two occasions, but has been brief and has been followed by continuing CTT support. There is little doubt that this client has benefited from a reduction in the number and length of admissions, despite the seriousness and enduring nature of her problem. Importantly, the Mental Health Act has not had to be used for some years, and one might suggest that the availability of intensive treatment at an early stage could have contributed to this.

Another example was the case of a young woman, Ms A, who was being assessed under the Mental Health Act at the request of her GP. She was in an extreme state of anxiety, and was thought to be suffering from agitated depression. She was not sleeping, her mood was deteriorating and she was pacing about her parents' home continually. She was in a state of extreme and disproportionate anxiety about her job. Her carers were no longer able to cope alone, and the GP and the psychiatrist were of the opinion that admission to hospital was unavoidable, a suggestion to which Ms A vehemently objected. It was clear that some form of action was required. A member of the CTT was present at the assessment, and was able to offer to visit the following day (a Saturday) and daily thereafter, leading to a palpable lessening of tension in the situation, and more especially, in the client. A further outcome was that the CPN was able, throughout her work with Ms A, to help pinpoint the real focus of the problem, which had not been evident at the outset. Thus admission, and probably a legal detention, was avoided.

Conclusion

A slightly sobering point to remember, despite the undoubtedly positive impact of the home treatment service in this area, is the fact that Mental Health Act assessments continue to rise in the county as well as nationally (Wall et al 1999). As seen in the results, however, the rise was slower in the area with the home treatment service.

As has been suggested in this study, a home treatment service can offer a real alternative to some people in some circumstances. This should lend weight to attempts to establish or extend such provision, in the spirit of advancing client choice and satisfaction, and the principles of community care in general. Continuing efforts in this direction could focus on extending home treatment in terms of the length of time spent with the client at each visit, and on developing more intermediate sorts of care, with the structure and safety of a 'holding' environment (Bion in Grotstein 1981).

If early referral and home treatment can lead to a lessening of the distress and disruption caused by a mental health crisis, and a

Mental Health Act assessment, then this in itself is a powerful argument for promoting it. Any forthcoming changes in mental health legislation will not alter this (HMSO 1999). The widest possible range of choices open to workers and clients makes the duty of the ASW to find the least restrictive alternative more realistic, meaningful, thoughtful and respectful, and shows a genuine commitment to community care. Admission under the Mental Health Act, if unavoidable, is more likely to be a genuine last resort, and can be carried out, in the words of one experienced ASW, '. . . with a slightly lighter heart'.

References

Barnes M, Bowl R, Fisher M (1990) Sectioned: Social Services and the 1983 Mental Health Act. London: Routledge.

Bateson G (ed) (1974) Perceval's narrative: A Patient's Account of His Psychosis 1830–1832 in Showalter E (1987) The Female Malady. London: Virago.

Bean P, Mounser P (1993) Discharged From Mental Hospitals. London: MIND.

Creed F (1995) Evaluation of community treatments for acute psychiatric illness. In: Tyrer P, Creed F (eds) Community Psychiatry in Action. Cambridge: Cambridge University Press.

Dean C, Phillips J, Gadd E, Joseph M, England S (1993) Comparison of community based service with hospital based service for people with acute, severe psychiatric illness. British Medical Journal 307:473–476.

Dunn LM (2001) Mental Health Act Assessments: Does a Community Treatment Team Make a Difference? International Journal of Social Psychiatry. Awaiting publication.

Fenton FR, Tessier L, Struening EL (1979) A comparative trial of home and hospital psychiatric care. Archives of General Psychiatry 36:1073–1079.

Flannigan C, Glover G, Wing J, Lewis S, Bebbington P, Feeney S (1984) Inner London collaborative audit of admission in two health districts. III: Reasons for acute admission to psychiatric wards. British Journal of Psychiatry 165:750–759.

Foucault M (1967) Madness and Civilization – a history of insanity in the age of reason. London: Tavistock.

Fulop NJ, Koffman J, Carson S, Robinson A, Pashley D, Coleman K (1996) Use of acute beds: a point prevalence study in North and South Thames regions. Journal of Public Health Medicine 18(2):207–216.

Glover GR, Robin E, Emami J, Rabsheibani R (1995) Mental Illness Needs Index (MINI) (computer program).

Grotstein JS (1981) Splitting and Projective Identification. New York: Aronson.

Hatfield B, Mohamad H, Huxley P (1992) The 1983 Mental Health Act in five local authorities: a study of the practice of approved social workers. International Journal of Social Psychiatry 38(3):189–207.

Herts County Council (1996) Locality Planning Information Database Version 2 (computer program).

Hertfordshire Social Services (1997) Report of the work of the Approved Social Worker. Herts Social Services.

HMSO (1999) Reform of the Mental Health Act 1983. Proposals for Consultation. London: HMSO.

Holloway F (1995) Home treatment as an alternative to acute psychiatric admission: a discussion. In: Tyrer P, Creed F (eds) Community Psychiatry in Action. Analysis and Prospects. Cambridge: Cambridge University Press.

Hoult J, Rosen A, Reynolds I (1984) Community orientated treatment compared to psychiatric hospital orientated treatment. Social Science and Medicine 18(11):1005–1010.

Marks I, Connolly J, Muijen M, Audini B, McNamee G, Lawrence R (1994) Home-based versus hospital-based care for people with serious mental illness. British Journal of Psychiatry 165:179–194.

Merson S, Tyrer P, Onyett S et al (1992) Early intervention in psychiatric emergencies: a controlled clinical trial. Lancet 339:1311–1314.

Pasamanick B, Scarpitti F, Dinitz S (1967) Schizophrenics in the Community. New York: Appleton-Century-Crofts.

Simpson C, Seager C, Robertson J (1993) Home-based care for patients with severe mental illness: a randomised controlled trial. British Journal of Psychiatry 162:239–243.

Stein I, Test MA (1980) Alternative to mental hospital treatment. I. Conceptual model, treatment program, and clinical evaluation. Archives of General Psychiatry 37:392–397.

Turner T, Ness M, Imison C (1992) Mentally disordered persons found in public places - diagnostic and social aspects of police referrals (Section 136). Psychological Medicine 22:765–774.

Wall S, Hotopf S, Wessely S, Churchill R (1999) Trends in the use of the Mental Health Act: England 1984–96. British Medical Journal 318:1520–1521.

WHCH (1997) Dacorum Community Treatment Team – Admissions, Activities and Assessments. St Albans: West Herts Community (NHS) Trust.

CHAPTER 6

Intensive home treatment for individuals with suicidal ideation

NEIL BRIMBLECOMBE

Summary

Key issues in assessing and providing intensive home treatment to clients with suicidal ideation are discussed, including clinical guidelines and a study of the relationship between suicidal ideation, home treatment and admission.

Suicide and mental health services

Suicide is a key issue in modern day mental health practice. The Health of the Nation initiative (DoH 1993) defined suicide as an area for priority action, both among the general public and among clients of mental health services. This emphasis has recently been reiterated in the National Service Framework for Mental Health (Department of Health 1999). This followed a rise in suicide rates with concern particularly being expressed in relation to increases in young men and other groups, such as young women of Asian descent.

Because of the frequency with which risk to self is cited as a reason for referral for hospital admission (Flannigan et al 1984), with suicidal ideation potentially acting as a 'talisman' in gaining admission (Elwood 1999), this has inevitably become an important issue for intensive home treatment (IHT) services offering alternatives to admission. Such services have recently increased in numbers and shall continue to do so (See Orme, Chapter 2).

IHT teams are typically extended-hours services (some covering 24 hours a day), offering a rapid initial response to referrals and able to provide frequent home visits to follow up. A common goal for such teams is to prevent admissions whenever possible by offering IHT as an alternative, and facilitate early discharge from inpatient areas through the same means. Teams commonly consist of community mental health nurses, psychiatrists, support workers and occasionally social workers and/or occupational therapists. The existence of these teams allows greater client choice, helps to avoid some of the negative effects of hospital admission and allows beds to be more easily available for those most in need of the high levels of supervision and relatively protected environment that can be provided to inpatients.

Concerns about increased risk

Concerns have been expressed that increasing the focus on providing community-based care will increase risk (Morgan 1992). Research into services offering IHT as an alternative to admission has yet to produce significant evidence to support such fears. The majority of studies of the performance of such services have found similar or, occasionally, lower suicide rates in those services providing extended-hours intensive community-based care. A Cochrane Review of five randomised controlled studies into 'crisis' home treatment services compared with 'standard' hospital-focused care showed no significant differences in suicide rates (Joy, Adams and Rice 1999).

Frequently there have been no deaths at all in studies (Langsley et al 1969, Stein and Test 1980, Hoult et al 1984, Tufnell et al 1988, Dean et al 1993, Minghella et al 1998, Cohen 1999). This at least partly illustrates how relatively uncommon an event suicide is, even in the acutely ill.

One study which did originally report a higher rate of suicide was that of the Daily Living Programme in Southwark, where three suicides (and a murder) were initially reported among their 92 clients, as opposed to two deaths from self-harm in a hospital-focused care control group of 97 clients (Marks et al 1994). Subsequently it emerged that there had been a further 18 deaths in other in- and outpatient services in the area, suggesting very high rates across all services (Connolly et al 1996).

Although it is hard to produce absolute proof that community-focused services (at least in an intensive form) are as safe as traditional services, it is clear that admission to hospital is no guarantee that suicide will be prevented. For those individuals committing suicide who had contact with mental health services in the year before their deaths, 13% of suicides actually took place while they were inpatients. A further 28% took place within 3 months of discharge from hospital (Appleby et al 1997).

Suicidal ideation and home treatment services

With most IHT services set up specifically to provide an alternative to psychiatric admission, it is to be expected that a significant proportion of referrals received will be of people presenting as a risk to self.

So what is the evidence so far? A Welsh intensive support team for community mental health team clients at risk of readmission found the most frequent reason for referral to their service was 'suicidal behaviour' (Coleman et al 1998), and in North Birmingham one of the most common reasons for clients being taken on for home treatment was that of 'risk of self-harm' (Minghella et al 1998). In West Herts the most frequent reason given for admission from an IHT team, once home treatment had started, was 'risk to self', at 50% ($n = 16$) of all such admissions (Brimblecombe and O'Sullivan 1999). In terms of what proportion of home treatment clients present with suicidal ideas, 55% ($n = 23$) of clients of the Manchester Home Option Service were seen as such (Harrison et al 1999). Interestingly this was a higher proportion than found in inpatient areas (32%, $n = 11$). The authors suggest that either there is a heightened sensitivity to identifying suicidal ideation in the home treatment team (they were using a detailed risk assessment tool), or home treatment services may be especially well suited to caring for those with suicidal ideation.

Suicidal ideation and the West Herts community treatment teams

In North West Herts two community treatment teams (CTTs) have been set up as part of the general shift towards community-focused care over the last few years. These services are additional to those provided by the four community mental health teams in the area, whose CPNs and social workers work on a more traditional 9 a.m.–5 p.m, Monday–Friday pattern, with an emphasis on long-term support, treatment and monitoring for those with, mostly, long-term severe mental illness. The CTTs, however, are available from 9 a.m. to 11 p.m. 7 days a week and specifically offer a service to those with severe, acute mental health problems who might otherwise require inpatient admission. Both teams consist of seven RMNs and a support worker, with psychiatrist support, covering a combined population of approximately 250 000.

Clients of the team are visited from several times a week to several times a day. The CTT may be involved for periods as short as a day or for as long as several months. Involvement continues until the client's needs can be adequately met by the more limited input available from other community resources, such as CPNs, day centres or psychiatric outpatients.

A study (Brimblecombe 2000) was carried out over a 12 month period. Details were recorded for all assessments carried out by the two community treatment teams of individuals referred in the community as potentially requiring admission. The Scale for Suicide Ideation (Beck et al 1979) was completed immediately after assessment unless this was impossible because the client was unwilling or unable to answer questions. The SSI is a 19 item instrument designed to quantify and assess suicidal ideation. Each item is scored on an increasing level of intensity from 0 to 2. Questions assess general attitude towards living, e.g. 'wish to live', as well as actions specifically related to suicidal intent, e.g. 'suicide note'. The measure has been claimed to be a reliable and valid instrument and has been widely used in research as a measure of 'suicidality' (Range and Knott 1997). In this study the first four items of the scale were used as a screening tool, the rest of the scale only being completed if a positive score was found on these initial items (Miller et al 1986). Training sessions were provided for staff before the study began in order to improve inter-rater reliability with the scale.

An examination was made of the frequency with which clients were rated as having suicidal ideation (i.e. scoring above 0 on the SSI) in relation to which service they received following assessment (Table 6.1). In 19 cases it was not possible to complete the SSI, usually because the client was not able or willing to answer questions.

There was a statistically significant difference ($\chi^2 = 56.20$, $df = 2$, $p < 0.001$) between the frequency for each outcome dependent on the presence of suicidal ideation. Of those admitted 46% were rated as experiencing suicidal ideation, compared with one-third of those

Table 6.1: Outcomes with and without suicidal ideation

Status after assessment	SSI score = 0 % (n)	SSI score > 0 % (n)
Admitted	53.7 (51)	46.3 (44)
Home treatment	66.7 (190)	33.3 (95)
Neither admission nor home treatment	89.8 (202)	10.2 (23)
Total	73.2 (443)	26.8 (162)

given home treatment and just one-tenth of those given neither home treatment nor admission. Although suicidal ideation was clearly related to an increased likelihood of admission, it was also clear that such ideation far from automatically led to admission, with 73% of such individuals not being admitted and 59% being given IHT as an alternative to admission.

Even when an admission at assessment took place of someone with a positive score, this was not necessarily always the direct cause of admission. When admitting staff were asked about the most important reason for admission in such cases, 23% (n = 10) of cases were reasons other than 'risk to self', most common being 'client's preference' (n = 6). Also, 25% (n = 12) of those admitted because of 'risk to self' (13% of all admissions) had SSI scores of 0, indicating that suicidal intent was not the important factor in the perceived risk; rather this was more likely due to non-deliberate risky behaviour, e.g. disinhibition or wandering late at night. This is important as it shows that the language used to categorise reasons for admission can give misleading impressions.

Conclusions from the West Herts study

There were limitations to this study, e.g. raters were not blind to outcomes, the validity of the SSI is limited in that positive scores do not always directly relate to suicidal ideas, and there may be variations between geographical areas in the frequency and nature of clients with suicidal ideas. With these caveats in mind, what conclusions can be drawn from these findings?

The majority of those presenting with suicidal ideation (as measured by the SSI) can avoid admission with the availability of an IHT team. However, a significant minority, often with higher total scores, will require admission no matter how comprehensive the community resources. A proportion of this group will actually be admitted, not so much because of direct concerns about their suicidal intent, but rather because they do not wish to work with the home treatment team. When individuals with suicidal ideation are taken on for home treatment a proportion of them will subsequently require admission (as with IHT clients with other problems).

Assessment and interventions

Having established that IHT services are frequently likely to work with individuals with suicidal ideation, a range of actions and considerations are described below which are important in providing care in a relatively safe and effective manner (Brimblecombe 1998). The categories described will inevitably overlap and other interventions may be required dependent on individual need and circumstance.

General assessment

Assessment can be seen as consisting of several stages.

The point of referral

In order to successfully access a service offering rapid assessment, suitable criteria must be met. Although there is likely to be a range of means of access to different services, there will almost invariably be a process of filtering to ensure that services see an appropriate client group. Whatever the stated criteria of a service, someone presenting with active suicidal ideation is likely to meet them. A process is required that attempts to elicit the possible presence of such ideas from the referrer. With all referrals, referrers should always be asked about evidence of such a risk. Demographic information, such as gender, age and previous history may also suggest an increased possibility of suicidal risk. Clearly the job of filtering referrals requires considerable skill and knowledge of risk factors, as well as assertiveness in declining referrals which are not urgent.

As with all assessments, it is important to gather whatever information is available before assessment (Brown 1998). Although there may be certain advantages in meeting a client without preconceptions, these are outweighed by the need to ascertain previous stressors, risks and treatment which may not always be ascertainable at any face to face assessment.

Initial assessment

In some cases (basically if there appears to be immediate risk to the potential client or others) it is clear that this must be done rapidly. Any service that hopes to intervene with those with suicidal ideation clearly needs to be able to respond quickly where there is evidence of immediate risk. Such services commonly set themselves target response times of 1–2 hours, with 4 hours as the maximum.

The assessment needs to be as full as possible, taking into account the social systems of the referred client as well as just looking for psychopathology (see Chapter 4). It is often useful to assess in the presence of others who know the client well, especially if the client already has a CPN or social worker. A psychiatrist and nurse constitute the assessing team, with the advantage this brings of providing a range of skills and experience (Sutherby and Szmukler 1995). Although broad principles of assessing those with suicidal ideation are well established, a greater focus than usual may be required in relation to several issues:

- the client's stated willingness, motivation or ability to work with the home treatment team (Harrison et al 1999)
- other supports available in the home setting
- ability to begin to form some sort of rapport.

In terms of risk assessment an approach is required which takes into account both individual characteristics and demographic features.

Although the assessment of risk in relation to self-harm is a difficult undertaking, detailed and informed attempts must be made (Gunnell and Frankel 1994). There is a huge range of literature concerning risk factors in relation to suicide, but prospective studies of suicide scales have not been successful at predicting short-term risk (Pokorney 1983, Beck et al 1985). Identified factors may have a statistically significant link with subsequent death, but are poorly correlated; that is, the presence of any, or several, of these factors in any individual indicates only a low percentage of chance of suicide. Even then, the chance of this happening may be over a period of years rather than in the short term which is the immediate concern of any IHT.

Undoubtedly, the clearest statistical predictor of future behaviour is past behaviour. Yet general knowledge that an individual has a history of self-harm is not enough to accurately target those most at risk. For example, the risk of suicide in the year following a suicide attempt is only 1 in 100 (although this is still 100 times that of the rest of the population) (Hawton 1987).

In addition to general demographic features, what is required is person-specific information concerning past events, including the contextual circumstances of previous self-harm and its dangerousness, both in medical terms and in the perception of the client. There is then a need to relate previous circumstances to the current situation (Vinestock 1996).

- What is the same, what is different?
- Are social supports more or less available?
- Has the client developed new ways of coping?
- Are there more or fewer factors making suicide a more or less likely action (e.g. physical illness, having young children)?

The key action in any assessment of suicidal ideation is to discuss the issue with the client. Avoiding the subject is not an alternative, and there is no evidence that raising the issue will instil the idea where it did not previously exist (Hyman 1994).

Ongoing reassessment

Clearly, although the initial assessment must attend very closely to aspects of risk, what is equally important is that assessment cannot be a 'one off'. On every subsequent visit there needs to be further reassessment, again with particular focus on the area of risk originally identified. IHT staff need to pay a good deal of attention to the manner in which all contacts are recorded, both to improve communication within the team and because, realistically, they must always be able to demonstrate that those actions that should have been carried out were carried out.

Suicides of clients in mental health services often take place during an apparent period of clinical improvement (Morgan 1992). The close daily monitoring of suicidal ideation is essential as part of ongoing risk assessment. Fears that persistently focusing on suicide may be detrimental are unsupported, and there is some limited evidence that self-monitoring may actually help decrease suicidal ideation (Clum and Curtin 1993). Certainly through close monitoring staff have the opportunity to help the client make links between any environmental and social changes around them and changes in their own levels of suicidal ideation.

Statement of intent

A starting point of working with a client at home must, almost invariably, be some type of statement from the client that they will not commit suicide. Morgan et al (1994) even suggest a written 'contract' to this effect. However, to request such a broad undertaking is often too great a demand. It may invite either dishonesty and consequent risk, or a tendency for clients to be admitted if they do not feel able to make such an extended commitment. The choice of question can usefully be more focused, e.g. 'can you say that you will not attempt to harm yourself before our next visit at 4 o'clock this afternoon?'. This type of question may be repeated every time a client is seen, even if this is three times a day. It may be useful to explain to the client at the beginning of a period of care that every time they are visited the IHT worker will need to ask them how they are coping with ideas of harming themselves, or if they have any current plans of killing or harming themselves. Keeping goals of staying alive minimal and achievable in terms of time reduces pressure on both the client and the worker. The ability of the individual client to be able to cooperate with the care offered is a vital factor in being able to successfully offer home treatment (Harrison et al 1999).

Identifying and utilising social supports

Relatives and friends are an important source of support to many at times of crisis. IHT workers can attempt to make these forms of support more systematic and integrate them into the overall plan of care. Timed visits to, or from, friends, or a relative popping in during the middle of the day, can make a substantial difference to an individual struggling, at times, to control impulses to self-harm. However, it is important that no one be forced into a role which they either do not wish for or are too anxious to be able to fulfil. Giving time to carers to discuss their fears and raise queries can make a substantial difference in their own perceived ability to cope and be supportive to the named client.

Conversely carers, friends and relatives do not always act in ways beneficial to the client; indeed, many depressive episodes are inextricably linked to interpersonal problems or pathological relationships. In such cases, where advice or perhaps trying to remove the patient from the home setting for short periods (for example in day care), is not successful, then hospital admission may be the only recourse. Of course, physically removing someone from an interpersonal difficulty may only be a short-term answer, and is one of the reasons that working through problems in situ is often a better approach.

Available resources

In addition to carers, it is often useful to ensure that the client has a list of those other resources easily available. The most important resource is likely to be the IHT service itself, so telephone numbers, key names and an invitation to contact whenever necessary should always be given. The Bradford Home Treatment Team even provides telephoneless clients with mobile telephones to make this easier (see Bracken, Chapter 7). Short-term coping strategies can usefully be discussed in the event of any brief delay between the client attempting to contact the IHT and any response. If services do not cover 24 hours, reminders should be given of resources outside working hours – the duty GP, the Samaritans, and direct contact with the inpatient units. Clients fearful of their own impulses are often reassured by knowing that they could refer themselves for assessment at inpatient facilities out of IHT team hours.

Rapport

A tremendously important event that needs to take place during assessment is the initial forming of rapport and starting to develop a relationship. Without some rapport the chances of successfully applying any of the other interventions described here are poor. It is perhaps unsurprising that services have, at times, noted that working with individuals with marked personality disorders can be difficult and they may be more likely to require inpatient care (Brimble-combe and O'Sullivan 1999, Bracken and Cohen 1999). Such individuals often show an inability to negotiate and form supportive relationships with others, which can be seen as a basic prerequisite for working with individuals with suicidal ideation in a non-hospital setting. Additionally, of course, in order to be able to work with anyone with suicidal ideation in the community it is essential that the worker believes that the client will be fairly honest with them.

Honesty and negotiating

Part of the relationship building will involve the worker being honest with the client, especially about concerns, e.g. that the client may take their own life, or in terms of discussing the likely speed of recovery. Negotiation also plays an important part in the assessment and in deciding what happens next. Home treatment workers are often in a position where essentially they are offering something to the client in terms of a service and support, in return for which the client is offering to stay alive for long enough to give workers an opportunity to help them. Part of that negotiation may also require substantial changes in the way the client deals with their everyday life. They may be asked to attend day centres, drink less or take a plethora of medications – essentially all of this relies on their agreement and at least a passive acceptance of the need for these changes.

Availability of means to self-harm

Home treatment workers are likely to spend much time in considering issues of availability of the means to self-harm. It is self-evident that anyone with sufficient determination can take their own life, including, of course, a patient in an inpatient psychiatric unit. However, most individuals with ideas of self-harm do not have such clear resolve. Many are at risk on impulse rather than clear and planned intent. Many are clear that they have only ever considered one means of killing themselves, most commonly through overdose.

This specific risk can be minimised by paying attention to both the type and the quantity of any medication provided (Appleby et al 1999). Clearly medication may potentially be of value to many clients with suicidal ideation, for example in terms of treating moderate to severe depression, alleviating psychotic symptoms, or temporarily helping reduce distressing sleep disturbance. Henry (1996) concludes that as many as 50% of those prescribed an antidepressant who commit suicide do so by an overdose of that antidepressant. Tricyclic antidepressants are valuable psychotropic drugs, especially with their sedating properties. However, overdose levels are often low. Serotonic specific re-uptake inhibitors (SSRIs) are significantly safer, but giving a month's prescription to anyone with a history or current thoughts of self-harm can be unwise and in some cases provocative. The benefits of medication must therefore be weighed against risk produced by injudicious prescribing.

IHT services, being able to visit frequently, may often be able to negotiate with the client to remove and hold supplies of their medication and sometimes administer this on a daily basis during the crisis period. Although this seems to be common practice, at least in the short term, it is, of course, potentially problematic in a couple of areas.

- It is perfectly clear that anyone with any mobility can go to the local pharmacy and buy sufficient supplies of drugs to commit suicide. Therefore any IHT worker must be clear that removing medication is a limited intervention, helpful only to those who are at risk from the most spontaneous and unplanned self-harm. In fact it appears, at times, to be more helpful as a symbolic indication of concern than as a practical way of preserving life.
- There is a risk that removing medication may also remove some of the client's sense of responsibility and encourage future acting out. This issue can most commonly be approached by explaining clearly that the intervention is a short-term one and as soon as the client and worker feel more confident, then the amount of medication held by the client can be increased, e.g. to two doses, then to two days, etc.

Psychological interventions

In terms of direct psychological interventions there are wide variations in individual needs. Generally however, a two-pronged focus may be useful in the period of greatest risk. Firstly, basic counselling skills of reflection and active listening are used to try and help the client express their feelings of distress, anger or hopelessness. This catharsis is useful, but should normally be linked to a focused practical problem-solving approach. This second approach focuses on identification of key stressors and discussion of strategies for reducing these or coping with them differently. Carers can sometimes also be involved in this process. The process of closely monitoring changes in levels of suicidal ideation can be used to help the client make links between events and mood changes (Clum and Curtin 1993).

'Timetabling'

A strategy which can frequently be utilised is to plan carefully with the client what they are doing for the next 24 hours or until the next visit by the team. This can be done in detail, making particular note of when they are alone or which times of the day are most likely to be vulnerable periods. Strategies of how to cope in these periods need to be addressed directly, e.g. 'what will you do if you have an urge to harm yourself when your wife is out shopping?'. The client may decide to keep busy during this vulnerable time with some chore, or may contract to telephone someone before self-harming; an IHT visit may be arranged for that time, or a different intervention can be planned based on the client's unique needs and resources.

Day care can be useful in several ways: as a means of not being alone, as a way of having an opportunity to engage in distracting and rewarding activities, to combat loneliness, etc. Some services, such as those in West Herts, are able to access acute day care specifically set up to offer such a facility, where transport is provided, staffing levels are relatively high and there is close liaison with the IHT team.

Admission

A vital aspect of being able to care for any individual in the community is the ability to have relatively easy access to inpatient areas when this is necessary. As mentioned above, IHT teams may expect to admit anywhere between 11% (Bracken and Cohen 1999) and 34% (Minghella et al 1998) of clients after home treatment has started. Analysis of admissions suggests that up to 50% may be admitted because of concerns about risk to self, mostly due to risk of suicide (Brimblecombe and O'Sullivan 1999). These admissions can often be of just a few days' duration and help the client through a particular crisis. IHT clients can usefully be made aware that if the situation deteriorates in the community then they can be admitted to hospital. This message gives reassurance and avoids a need for acting out in a self-destructive way for those who feel a need for some temporary asylum care. An equally important message (for workers as well as the client) is that admission does not mean 'failure'. Admission is simply a different way to try and help meet a client's immediate needs.

Recording

A key worker should be appointed from within the team who is responsible for maintaining a detailed care plan. As one worker alone cannot usually provide all the care, owing to the frequency of visits required and the possibility of extra visits in emergencies, the care plan must be clear and concise enough for others to be able to refer to and follow. Aims and interventions that are stated in simple behavioural terms are more easily applied, and progress can be assessed by anyone who needs to see the client (Brimblecombe 1995).

The process of defining and setting goals is an important one in itself. The sense of achievement gained through working towards a series of minimal, achievable but meaningful goals can be an important contribution to rebuilding the client's self-confidence (Weakland et al 1974).

It is always vital that details of assessments, subsequent events and care plans be meticulously kept. Clearly in dealing with this client group there is always an element of risk; even the most thorough assessment cannot absolutely guarantee against future suicide. It is therefore essential that records clearly demonstrate the thoroughness of the care given. This is especially important as IHT services are still generally novel and any negative incidents may attract greater scrutiny than when they occur in more routine services (Connolly et al 1996).

Withdrawal

The issue of the withdrawal of home treatment team support is always an important one. Such teams will normally remain involved only long enough to help the client improve to the stage where other resources are able to provide adequate levels of care. It is vital that the resources of such teams are able to be freed to provide the rapid response and high input levels needed by those newly, severely ill; however; the loss of a service that has been so involved can be a difficult process for the client.

This potential problem is approached in a number of ways.

- First, information should be given early on, often at the point of assessment, that the home treatment team is likely to be involved for only a relatively short time. A written leaflet summarising the aims and methods of a service may be useful here.
- Second, the process of reducing input is normally a gradual one and part of a negotiated process. The number of visits may be reduced over a period of weeks, or telephone contacts may gradually replace home visits. Issues of loss must be acknowledged and discussed.
- Third, the ensuring of adequate follow-up from other resources must be carefully addressed, with close links maintained with community mental health teams, outpatients, clinics and other agencies.
- Fourth, the client can be made aware of the availability of the IHT team in the future should things get worse again.

Conclusions

Evidence now clearly demonstrates that home treatment services are able to provide care for many individuals with suicidal ideation without the need for hospital admission. Despite the difficulties inherent in this endeavour, there is no evidence that suicide rates are higher in such services than in those relying more on hospital admission. Further research is still required to investigate the link between admission and suicidal ideation in more detail. Surprisingly little exists so far. This is despite the high proportion of admissions (Flannigan et al 1984) and the large amount of mental health service resources taken up by individuals presenting with suicidal ideation.

Particular patterns of suicide may actually suggest an additional role for IHT teams. The National Confidential Inquiry into Suicide and Homicide by People with Mental Illness (Appleby et al 1999) noted the high levels of suicide in the month following discharge from inpatient units, and in particular in the first week. Although there can only be speculation about the cause of this, two possible actions may be suggested.

- Admissions should only take place when absolutely necessary. Home treatment provides greater opportunities for the resolution, in situ, of social problems causing or aggravating mental health problems and also allows for a more graduated withdrawal of services once the acute episode has improved.

- Where admission is definitely required, IHT teams can provide relatively intensive short-term input to ease the transition from hospital back to the community and to allow for greater levels of monitoring of resurgent suicide risk than traditional community services could provide.

References

Appleby L, Shaw J, Amos T et al (1997) National Confidential Inquiry into Suicide and Homicide by People with Mental Illness: Progress Report. London: Department of Health.

Appleby L, Shaw J, Amos T et al (1999) Safer services. The National Confidential Inquiry into Suicide and Homicide by People with Mental Illness. London: HMSO.

Beck AT, Kovacs M, Weissman A (1979) Assessment of suicidal intention: The Scale for Suicide Ideation. Journal of Consulting and Clinical Psychology 47(2):343–352.

Beck A, Steer RA, Kovacs M, Garrison B (1985) Hopelessness and eventual suicide: a 10-year prospective study of patients hospitalized with suicidal ideation. American Journal of Psychiatry 142:559–563.

Bracken P, Cohen B (1999) Home treatment in Bradford. Psychiatric Bulletin 23:349–352.

Brimblecombe N (1995) The use of brief therapy as part of the nursing care plan. Nursing Times 91(35):34–35.

Brimblecombe N (1998) Supporting clients with suicidal impulses in the community. Nursing Times 94(10): 49–51.

Brimblecombe N (2000) Suicidal ideation, home treatment and admission. Mental Health Nursing 20(1):22–26.

Brimblecombe N, O'Sullivan G (1999) Diagnosis, assessments and admissions from a community treatment team. Psychiatric Bulletin 23:72–74.

Brown T (1998) Psychiatric emergencies. Advances in Psychiatric Treatment 4:270–276.

Clum GA, Curtin L (1993) Validity and reactivity of a system of self-monitoring suicide ideation. Journal of Psychopathology and Behavioral Assessment 15(4):375–385.

Cohen BMZ (1999) Innovatory forms of evaluation for new crisis services. Science, Discourse and Mind 1(1):12–31.

Coleman M, Donnelly P, Davies A, Brace P (1998) Evaluating intensive support in community mental health care. Mental Health Nursing 18(5):8–11.

Connolly J, Marks I, Lawrence R, McNamee G, Muijen M (1996) Observations from community care for serious mental illness during a controlled study. Psychiatric Bulletin 20:3–7.

Dean C, Phillips J, Gadd E, Joseph M, England S (1993) Comparison of community based service with hospital based service for people with acute, severe psychiatric illness. British Medical Journal 307:473–476.

DoH (1993) The Health of the Nation. Key Area Handbook: Mental Illness. Heywood: Department of Health.

DoH (1999) National Service Framework: Mental Health. DoH: London.

Elwood PY (1999) Characteristics of admissions considered inappropriate by junior psychiatrists. Psychiatric Bulletin 23:34–37.

Flannigan C, Glover G, Wing J, Lewis S, Bebbington P, Feeney S (1984) Inner London collaborative audit of admission in two health districts. III: Reasons for acute admission to psychiatric wards. British Journal of Psychiatry 165:750–759.

Gunnell D, Frankel S (1994) Prevention of Suicide: Aspirations and evidence. British Medical Journal 308: 1227–1233.

Harrison J, Poynton A, Marshall J, Gater R, Creed F (1999) Open all hours: extending the role of the psychiatric day hospital. Psychiatric Bulletin 23:400–404.

Hawton K (1987) Assessment of suicide risk. British Journal of Psychiatry 150:145–153.

Henry JA (1996) Suicide risk and antidepressant treatment. Journal of Psychopharmacology 10(suppl 1):39–40.

Hoult J, Rosen A, Reynolds I (1984) Community orientated treatment compared to psychiatric hospital orientated treatment. Social Science and Medicine 8(11):1005–1010.

Hyman SE (1994) The suicidal patient. In: Hyman SE, Tesar GE (eds) Manual of Psychiatric Emergencies, 3rd edn. Boston: Little Brown.

Joy CB, Adams CE, Rice K (1999) Crisis intervention for people with severe mental illnesses (Cochrane Review). In: The Cochrane Library 1. Oxford: Update Software.

Langsley DG, Flomenhaft K, Machotka P (1969) Followup evaluation of family crisis therapy. American Journal of Orthopsychiatry 39(5):753–759.

Marks IM, Connolly J, Muijen M, Audini B, McNamee G, Lawrence RE (1994) Home-based versus hospital-based care for people with serious mental illness. British Journal of Psychiatry 165:179–194.

Miller IW, Norman WH, Dow MG, Bishop SB (1986) The modified Scale for Suicidal Ideation: reliability and validity. Journal of Consulting and Clinical Psychology 54(5):724–725.

Minghella E, Ford R, Freeman T, Hoult J, McGlynn P, O'Halloran P (1998) Open All Hours. 24-hour response for people with mental health emergencies. London: Sainsbury Centre for Mental Health.

Morgan G (1992) Suicide prevention. Hazards on the fast lane to community care. British Journal of Psychiatry 160: 149–153.

Morgan G, Jones R, Wiltshire J (1994) Secondary Care. In: Jenkins R, Griffiths S, Wylie I, Hawton K, Morgan G, Tylee A (eds) The Prevention of Suicide. London: HMSO.

Pokorney AD (1983) Prediction of suicide in psychiatric patients. Archives of General Psychiatry 40:249–257.

Range LM, Knott EC (1997) Twenty suicide assessment instruments: evaluation and recommendations. Death Studies 21:25–28.

Sutherby K, Szmukler G (1995) Community assessment of crisis. In: Phelan M, Strathdee G, Thornicroft G (ed) Emergency Mental Health Services in the Community. Cambridge: Cambridge University Press.

Vinestock M (1996) Risk assessment. "A word to the wise"? Advances in Psychiatric Treatment 2:3–10.

Weakland JH, Fisch R, Watzlawick P, Bodin AM (1974) Brief Therapy: Focused problem resolution. Family Process 13(2):141–168.

CHAPTER 7

The radical possibilities of home treatment: postpsychiatry in action

Patrick J. Bracken

Summary

The relevance of current psychiatric views of people in distress is considered. The origins and themes of 'postpsychiatry' are outlined. A home treatment service working with a non-psychiatric approach is described.

It is an exciting time to work in the world of mental health. Never before have users of psychiatric services been so organised and so vocal. As a result, in Britain at least, possibilities for real dialogue between users and professionals have begun. Moreover, if one believes, as I do, that psychiatry is born of the institution, then the move to community care may signal the dawning of a new era. Our engagement with people in distress will be transformed if it becomes possible to leave the conceptual baggage of the psychiatric hospital behind. These developments offer the prospect of revolution rather than reform in mental health care, and the chance to move away from traditional psychiatry altogether. I am in favour of such a revolution, and I advocate a therapeutic framework that is based on the notion of postpsychiatry. The term 'postpsychiatry' was coined by myself and Phil Thomas and is used as the title for our regular column in the journal *Open Mind*. I will discuss the term later in this chapter, but basically it refers to a situation where psychiatry no longer dominates our understanding of states of madness and distress (Bracken and Thomas 1998).

In my opinion, home treatment offers a golden opportunity, allowing us not only to change the site of mental health care but also radically to rethink the nature of that care. On a bleaker note,

I believe that if we do not seize this opportunity there will be a danger that community care, including home treatment, will simply serve to facilitate the transfer of oppressive theories and practices from the hospital into people's own homes.

In the next section I discuss the cultural origins of psychiatry and indicate why I think this analysis has relevance to the development of home treatment services. I shall then introduce what I loosely call 'the postpsychiatry agenda'. In the third section I shall bring these ideas to bear on the development of home treatment and discuss how my colleagues and I have attempted to develop a service in Bradford which is not based on the framework of traditional psychiatry. The home treatment team did not set out to 'put postpsychiatry into prac-tice'. My argument is that in seeking to develop a genuine alternative to hospital psychiatry they have ended up with a style of intervention which resonates strongly with the notion of postpsychiatry.

This chapter is unashamedly theoretical. If we are to challenge oppressive practices and systems of 'care', then this needs to take place at a number of levels. Theoretical analysis is important if we are to deny psychiatry's defence of its powerful position through an assertion of its scientific credentials. Only through an analysis of the history of psychiatry and the role of the hospital in that history do we get a glimpse of the real possibilities of home treatment. (The reader who simply wishes to read about home treatment in Bradford could skip the first two sections.)

The birth of psychiatry

The ways in which we understand the history of psychiatry and the notion of mental illness were changed substantially through the work of the French historian and philosopher, Michel Foucault. Foucault argued that psychiatry's story of its own development, as a straight-forward science-based branch of medicine, was fundamentally mistaken (Foucault 1967). He sought to counter a history in which the emergence of psychiatry in the past 200 years was seen simply to represent the decline of superstition and the triumph of science. Instead, he argued that psychiatry became possible only in a particu-lar cultural framework, one opened up by the European Enlighten-ment and the 'age of reason'. For Foucault, psychiatry is a cultural product and consequently is dependent on certain culturally based assumptions about the nature of the self and the order of the world. It cannot claim universal truth or validity. Just as other cultures have articulated various spiritual understandings of madness based on background religious beliefs, psychiatry's account of madness is, likewise, based on background orientations and beliefs that are peculiar to modern western culture.

A central concern of the European Enlightenment was the importance of reason and its place in human affairs (Hampson 1968). Finding a path to true knowledge and certainty became the major issue for thinkers during the Enlightenment, and a guiding theme was the quest to replace religious revelation and systems of knowledge from the past with reason and science as the path to truth. Enlightenment meant a move from 'darkness' to 'light'. To achieve this, 'reason' would boldly have to give up its preoccupation with those things handed down in tradition.

The other preoccupation of European thought emerging from the Enlightenment, particularly on the continent, was with the human self and its depths. European thinkers became concerned with the 'inner voice' and the structures of subjectivity (Solomon 1988). This was seen in the Romantic movement's concern with imagination and the expression of emotion. Poets, novelists and others sought to explore the internal world of individuals, their thoughts and feelings, in a way not done before. Initially this was a reaction against the Enlightenment focus on reason, but the two concerns very much came together in the late nineteenth century in the phenomenology of Husserl and, of course, in the psychoanalysis of Freud. Freud's stated aim was to bring the light of reason and science to bear on the dark irrational forces of the unconscious world. In Foucault's history, the concept of a separate realm of 'mental illness' and the development of a technology to treat such 'illness' only became a possibility (and eventually a necessity) in a culture preoccupied with rationality, science, technology and the nature of the individual self.

On a more practical level, with its focus on reason and order, the Enlightenment spawned an era in which society sought to rid itself of all 'unreasonable' elements. As the historian Roy Porter writes:

> The Enlightenment endorsed the Greek faith in reason ('I think, therefore I am', Descartes had claimed). And the enterprise of the age of reason, gaining

authority from the mid-seventeenth century onwards, was to criticize, condemn and crush whatever its protagonists considered to be foolish or unreasonable. All beliefs and practices which appeared ignorant, primitive, childish or useless came to be readily dismissed as idiotic or insane, evidently the products of stupid thought-processes, or delusion and daydream. And all that was so labelled could be deemed inimical to society or the state – indeed could be regarded as a menace to the proper workings of an orderly, efficient, progressive, rational society (Porter 1987, pp. 14–15).

In Foucault's account, the emergence of the institutions in which 'unreasonable' people were to be housed was not in itself a 'progressive', or medical, venture. It was simply, and crudely, an act of social exclusion. He coined the term 'the Great Confinement'. Furthermore, he argued that it was only when such people had been both excluded and brought together that they became subject to the 'gaze' of medicine. According to Foucault, doctors were originally involved in these institutions in order to treat physical illness and to offer moral guidance. They were not there as experts in disorders of the mind. As time went on, the medical profession came to dominate in these institutions and doctors began to order and classify the inmates in more systematic ways. Roy Porter writes:

> Indeed, the rise of psychological medicine was more the consequence than the cause of the rise of the insane asylum. Psychiatry could flourish once, but not before, large numbers of inmates were crowded into asylums (Porter 1987, p. 17).

Medical superintendents of asylums gradually became psychiatrists, but they did not start out as such. Alongside the increasing hegemony of psychiatrists, the concept of mental illness became accepted. In other words, in this account, the profession of psychiatry and its associated technologies of diagnosis and treatment only became possible in the institutional arena opened up by an original act of social rejection. Perhaps this explains some of the stigma which has been attached to psychiatry and its patients, in spite of the former's protestations of its scientific credentials. Historically, psychiatry emerged to label those who had already been rejected and thus its diagnoses quickly became symbols of rejection in themselves.

Although a number of psychiatrists and historians have questioned various aspects of Foucault's account, and it has become increasingly clear that the story of psychiatry has varied greatly from country to country (Foucault's focus was on developments in France), nevertheless there is a general acceptance that his rejection of a simple 'progressivist' version of psychiatry's development is justified (Gordon 1990). I want to examine the challenges raised by this. These can be stated as a series of related questions:

- If psychiatry is the product of the institution, should we not question its ability to guide the sort of care we want to deliver in the post-institutional era?
- Can we imagine a different relationship between medicine and madness, different, that is, from the one forged in the asylums and hospitals of a previous age?
- Can we begin to imagine different forms of mental health care which do not rely on psychiatry at all?
- If psychiatry is the product of a culture preoccupied with rationality and the individual self, what sort of mental health care is appropriate in the postmodern, multicultural world in which many of these preoccupations are starting to lose their dominance?
- Is western psychiatry appropriate to cultural groups who do not share these preoccupations, but instead are focused on a spiritual ordering of the world and an ethical emphasis on the importance of family and community?
- How can we uncouple mental health care from the agenda of social exclusion, coercion and control to which it became bound in the last two centuries?

I believe that if we do not face up to these questions we are in danger of replicating the problems of institutional care in our community services. Indeed, there is evidence that this has already begun to happen with a number of assertive outreach services in the US. Relying on the traditional medical approach to understanding madness and distress, these services often see the administration of medication as their most important goal. Other service elements are used to engage users but only in a bid to ensure compliance. As a result, many users have complained that they experience these services as being as oppressive as traditional hospital psychiatry and have begun to campaign against them (Oaks 1998). The concept of home treatment is often allied with that of assertive outreach. The dangers are obvious. My argument is that we can avoid these dangers in home treatment only by committing ourselves to a radical examination of the philosophy underlying our practice. If we do not do so, we risk replicating institutional power structures and relationships between professionals and users in the community. At the time of writing, the British government is proposing the introduction of 'community treatment orders' which will mean that many users of services could be forced to take psychiatric drugs while living in the community. If home treatment teams do not work with a clear philosophy of care, they could find themselves being used simply to enforce these orders.

In the next section I shall explain what I mean by postpsychiatry and argue that this offers a framework through which we can imagine a very different direction for mental health work.

Postpsychiatry

By the term 'postpsychiatry' I am seeking to characterise a move beyond the old debates between psychiatry and antipsychiatry. The latter sought to show that psychiatry was repressive and based on a mistaken medical ideology. Antipsychiatrists wanted to liberate mental patients from its clutches (Bracken 1995). In turn, psychiatry condemned its opponents as being driven by ideology (Roth and Kroll 1986). Both approached madness as something to be accounted for, something to be written about and something for which therapy was needed. Both positions were united by the assumption that there could be a correct way of understanding madness. There was an assumption that the truth could, and should, be spoken about states of madness and distress. Both sides of the argument assumed that truth and ideology were mutually exclusive.

Postpsychiatry is about a different way of framing the issues. Unlike antipsychiatry and previous forms of critical psychiatry it does not, itself, propose new theories about madness but by a deconstruction of psychiatry seeks to open up spaces in which other, alternative, understandings of madness can assume a validity denied them by psychiatry. Crucially, it argues that the voices of service users and survivors should now be centre-stage. Similarly, postpsychiatry seeks to distance itself from the therapeutic implications of antipsychiatry. It does not propose any new form of therapy to replace the medical techniques of psychiatry. Antipsychiatry, especially as developed by R. D. Laing, proposed a modified version of psychoanalysis (based largely on existential philosophy) as an alternative to psychiatry. Others, writing under the heading of 'critical psychiatry', such as Ingleby and Kovel, also looked to different versions of psychoanalysis to frame their theories and practice (Ingleby 1980). Postpsychiatry sees the theories of Freud and other analysts as part of the problem, not the solution!

To use a spatial metaphor, postpsychiatry is not a place, a set of fixed ideas and beliefs. Instead, it is more like a set of orientations which together can help us move on from where we are now. It does not seek to prescribe an end point and does not argue that there are 'right' and 'wrong' ways of tackling madness.

The term 'postpsychiatry' obviously echoes other postmodernist debates and perhaps it would be wise to outline my understanding of postmodernism before describing the main elements of a postpsychiatry position. I am aware that the concept of 'postmodernism' and the related concept of 'modernism' are somewhat nebulous and highly contended. For myself, the term 'modernism' refers to a cultural idiom which had its origins in the age of reason, discussed above. In the post-Enlightenment period, western societies became increasingly focused on science and technology. Both capitalist and communist social orders followed this path. Modernism placed great faith in reason and order and proposed that all human problems would eventually yield to the advance of science. The term 'postmodernism' is often used to refer to a contemporary social, cultural and political condition, something we simply find ourselves in the midst of. In contrast to the serious endeavours of modernism, the postmodern condition is said to be characterised by superficiality and playfulness. However, I shall use the term more positively, to refer to a way of reflecting on the world and our place within it.

I do not believe that a postmodernist perspective undermines the validity of other critical perspectives, such as those derived from Marxist theory. In fact, I am sympathetic to the position of writers such as Jameson (1991) and Harvey (1989) who seek to understand the culture of postmodernism in terms of underlying transformations in the nature of capitalism. Instead, I am seeking to work with insights derived from postmodern theory to develop a theoretical framework which can support radical change in the area of mental health. However, I concur with Parker (1998) that there are dangers inherent in the postmodernist position. In the end, theory should serve practice, not the other way around, and our main task now is the transformation of mental health care. I agree with Fred Newman and Lois Holzman (1997) that when Marx is understood primarily as an advocate of 'revolutionary activity' there is no contradiction between Marxism and the insights of postmodernism. In this regard, his most important observation was that 'the philosophers have only interpreted the world, in various ways; the point is to change it' (Marx 1977, p. 123).

For me, postmodernism is about facing the contradictions and difficulties of our situation as human beings without recourse to a belief that there will always be true and false ways of understanding and correct and incorrect ways of acting and behaving. In many ways postmodernism raises more problems than it answers, but it can claim a higher degree of honesty than positions which continue to assert that they have the truth or have the right path to the truth.

Two elements of postmodernism are important to our discussion of psychiatry. The first concerns the discourse of ethics. Recent years have witnessed the emergence of a 'postmodern ethics'. Zygmund Bauman, who overtly embraces the concept of postmodernism, argues that the modernist search for codification, universality and foundations in the area of ethics was actually destructive of the moral impulse (Bauman 1993). He argues for a 'morality without ethics'. By this he means that morality has never been about simply following an ethical code. Indeed such codes have often stood in the way of moral behaviour. For Bauman, postmodernism is about confronting the real moral dilemmas which face us without recourse to the illusion that there will always be a rational, correct solution. Bauman argues that modernism was animated by a belief in 'the possibility of a non-ambivalent, non-aporetic ethical code' (the term aporia refers to a contradiction that cannot be overcome, one that results in a conflict that cannot be resolved). In contrast, he says:

> What the postmodern mind is aware of is that there are problems in human and social life with no good solutions, twisted trajectories that cannot be straightened up, ambivalences that are more than linguistic blunders yelling to be corrected, doubts which cannot be legislated out of existence, moral agonies which no reason-dictated recipes can soothe, let alone cure (Bauman 1993, p. 245).

Postmodern ethics is not about a situation where 'anything goes'. It is rather about facing the world without easy recourse to guiding codes or principles. It is about an acceptance that ambivalence and disorder are aspects of life which we should embrace, not just temporary difficulties that need to be overcome by further analysis, or the application of ever more structured ethical systems. In addition, for postmodernists the modernist and rationalistic attempt to render our moral issues in simple dichotomies of good and bad, right and wrong, has had disastrous consequences. For example, Bauman sees such dichotomies operating in the Holocaust. He argues that the Holocaust was not simply an aberration in the development of modern society, but instead can be understood as a product of an Enlightenment quest for an orderly society. He writes:

> The unspoken terror permeating our collective memory of the Holocaust . . . is the gnawing suspicion that the Holocaust could be more than an aberration, more than a deviation from an otherwise straight path of progress, more than a cancerous growth on the otherwise healthy body of the civilised society; that, in short, the Holocaust was not an antithesis of modern civilization and everything (or so we like to think) it stands for. We suspect (even if we refuse to admit it) that the Holocaust could merely have uncovered another face of the same modern society whose other, more familiar, face we so admire (Bauman 1989, p. 7).

The lesson to be learnt by professionals is clear: you do not have, and never will have, all the answers. And, furthermore, the answers that will be relevant and useful will not always come from protocols and codes. The implication of this is that there are areas of human life that professionals should not seek to order, because that ordering will have a down side, a set of effects which will not be seen in advance. From the postmodern perspective the difficulties of institutional psychiatry, such as those described some time ago by Erving Goffman (1991) and more recently by the Sainsbury Centre (1998), are not simply an aberration, the consequences of bad behaviour by a few individuals, to be eliminated by new codes of practice and new forms of therapy. From this perspective, they show up as essential aspects of the modernist attempt to control madness and distress. They are its 'other face'. Indeed, from the postmodernist viewpoint the search for ever more efficient therapies and codes of behaviour is part of the problem and can be expected to generate new forms of oppression and suffering.

The second element of postmodernism of importance to us here is its understanding of knowledge, and the question of truth. As mentioned above, postmodernism involves a rejection of the idea that the truth can ever be regarded as something independent, neutral and uninvolved. Foucault is perhaps the major voice in this area and his writings have started to have substantial effects on the ways in which we think about science, and in particular science relating to human experience and behaviour. My comments here will not be extensive. I simply wish to show the reader how Foucault's analysis leads to a very different understanding of what is involved in the notion of 'truth' when compared with past debates between psychiatry and antipsychiatry. For Foucault, it is simply a mistake to believe that knowledge and truth can ever be separated from ideology. His writing about truth emerges from his work on power and knowledge, in which he argues that traditional concepts of power, as something essentially repressive, cannot account for the many functions of power in modern society. In his book *Discipline and Punish* he argues that:

> We must cease once and for all to describe the effects of power in negative terms; it 'excludes,' it 'represses,' it 'censors,' it 'abstracts,' it 'masks,' it 'conceals.' In fact power produces; it produces reality, it produces domains of objects and rituals of truth. The individual and the knowledge that may be gained of him belong to this production (Foucault 1977, p. 194).

In this way, he argues that knowledge is the concrete manifestation of the positive functioning of power. Knowledge is inextricably associated with networks of power:

> power produces knowledge (and not simply by encouraging it because it is useful); . . . power and knowledge directly imply one another; . . . there is no power relation without the correlative constitution of a field of knowledge, nor any knowledge that does not presuppose and constitute at the same time power relations (Foucault 1977, p. 27).

Foucault attempted to get beyond the idea that there was truth on one side and ideology on the other. What is acceptable as 'the truth' and how that can be separated from 'the false' is dependent on assumptions about what is acceptable evidence and how that evidence can be used. These are elements of what he calls a field of knowledge. Such fields of knowledge are not free-floating but are controlled in many different ways. Powerful institutions of our society both create these fields of knowledge and also depend upon them. The world of mental health is an obvious example. Foucault's approach to reason and rationality can be seen to follow from this. For him there is no such thing as an independent, and objective, reason. Instead, there are many different rationalities, all tied to various power formations for their meaning and validity. For Foucault, being critical did not involve adopting a position of rational superiority over others. Rather it involved a demonstration of the contingent origins and contexts of all systems of knowledge. In doing this, and in showing how knowledge is always political and thus value-laden, Foucault worked to open up spaces where other, often marginalised and silenced, voices could be heard.

Postpsychiatry uses these insights from postmodernist thought to develop a new agenda for mental health work. There are no 'basic principles', set in stone. As mentioned above, there are a series of orientations which can be used to frame work in this area. These orientations are not mutually exclusive and there is overlap between them all. The following is a first attempt!

The acceptance of multiple realities

There is no single correct way of accounting for reality. There are, in fact, multiple realities. Scientific accounts of the natural and human world are not mistaken, but neither are they the 'final word'. Science represents one way of ordering our world; there are other ways. This is not to say that 'anything goes' and each perspective has equal validity. Each approach to understanding has to defend its own assumptions. However, what is being asserted here is that there is no neutral vantage point from where we can objectively judge which account has more validity than the others. Psychiatry has to demonstrate its worth; it is no longer enough simply to assert its scientific and medical credentials. Postpsychiatry proposes that psychiatry has substantially overestimated its value, downplayed its oppressiveness and oversold its benefits.

An emphasis on social, political and cultural context

We have seen above how in the Enlightenment period the individual self became the focus of many different discourses. Influenced by

Husserlian phenomenology and Freudian psychoanalysis, psychiatry has been almost entirely premised upon this focus. It has located madness and distress within the confines of individual minds and has sought systematically to decontextualise these phenomena. It has achieved this by locating its encounters with patients in hospitals and clinics and by a therapeutic focus on the individual, either through drug treatments or through psychotherapy. Its scientific self-understanding has rendered it unable to see how both its own theories and practices are based on assumptions generated within the surrounding culture and how the distress it encounters is always produced, shaped and understood within particular social, political and cultural environments. However, postpsychiatry seeks a contextualist understanding of madness and distress and places a great emphasis on an attempt to reveal its own assumptions and how these influence its practice. It tries to balance a medical understanding of human pain with a hermeneutic approach to interpreting suffering as always happening in an interpersonal world.

The primacy of ethics over knowledge

Knowledge is never free from values and political intent. All knowledge emerges from a position of interest. Psychiatry has sought to present itself as being based upon a disinterested scientific account of madness and distress. However, postpsychiatry accepts that an ethic of social exclusion has been built into the heart of the psychiatric enterprise. Psychiatry is premised upon the assumption that reason has a right – indeed a duty – to speak about madness. Psychiatry assumes that it is justified in its own attempt to describe, analyse and, ultimately, diagnose madness. Postpsychiatry believes that these are ethical assumptions which cry out to be exposed. Postpsychiatry seeks to begin with values and a debate about ethics and argues that the use of knowledge and technology should be a secondary event. Postpsychiatry seeks to end the monologue of reason about madness and opens up a space in which the positive value of madness is revealed.

There is a downside to modernism

As discussed above, postmodernism is very much about an acknowledgement that there is a dark side to the project of Enlightenment. In the twenty-first century, the advances of science and technology are no longer welcomed with open arms by a public who have grown sceptical about the 'good life' promised by these advances. Disasters in nuclear technology and worries about genetic engineering are the stuff of our daily news. The enterprise of categorising and labelling madness and distress also has its downside. Diagnoses such as schizophrenia carry a burden for every individual and family who receive them. Psychiatry has argued that this burden is due to 'ignorance' on behalf of the general public about the true nature of mental illness, and has sought to 'educate' the public about these illnesses. However, postpsychiatry rejects many of the categories used by psychiatry as unnecessary, mystifying and potentially harmful and seeks to develop ways of understanding and helping people without easy recourse to diagnostic labels (Bracken and Thomas 1999).

Questioning the project of psychotherapy

Postpsychiatry also seeks to problematise the concept of psychotherapy. Earlier debates between psychiatry and antipsychiatry often became, in practice, disputes between biological approaches and psychotherapy. Postpsychiatry does not see psychotherapy as entirely benign. Psychotherapy is itself a product of current cultural preoccupations with individual needs and desires. It is presented as a positive and harmless alternative to biological therapies and its proponents fail to acknowledge the values on which it is premised and the potential dangers of its use.

The move from modernism to postmodernism has been explained in terms of a shift from an economic order based on the priority of production to one based, instead, on consumption. In a culture dominated by consumption there is an ever-expanding drive to create more desires and needs within individuals. The logic of the current economic system involves an increasing exhortation to consume and to experience our lives in terms of needs to be filled by new products, new services or some new expert discourse. Nickolas Rose writes:

> Consumption requires each individual to choose from among a variety of products in response to a repertoire of wants that may be shaped and legitimated by advertising and promotion but must be experienced and justified as personal desires . . . the modern self is institutionally required to construct a life through the exercise of choice from among alternatives (Rose 1989, p. 227).

We are, according to Rose, 'obliged to be free'. Not only do we have to choose items to feed our desires, however, but also to choose our values from a range with an ever-decreasing 'shelf-life'. He suggests that one function of therapy is to assist this process. He argues that, to a significant degree, we are now governed (ironically) through our own individual quests for freedom and self-expression:

> Psychotherapeutics is linked at a profound level to the socio-political obligations of the modern self. The self it seeks to liberate or restore is the entity able to steer its individual path through life by means of the act of personal decision and the assumption of personal responsibility. It is the self freed from all moral obligations but the obligation to construct a life of its own choosing, a life in which it realizes itself . . . (Rose 1989, pp. 253–4).

Postpsychiatry does not reject therapy but refuses to see it as the alternative to psychiatry.

These are the basic tenets of a postpsychiatry perspective. This is a new idea and will develop with time. It is not the only way of thinking critically about psychiatry. The next section has a focus on practice. I shall describe the home treatment service in Bradford and suggest that this provides an example of what postpsychiatry could mean within the statutory sector.

Home treatment in Bradford

The home treatment service has been operational in Bradford since 1996. As mentioned above, the team did not set out to work with a postpsychiatry perspective but, I will suggest, in attempting to develop a genuine alternative to hospitalisation for people with mental health crises, over time it has developed a style of work which is broadly in tune with the theoretical orientation I have tried to develop above. We have worked to move beyond the logic of traditional psychiatry but do not assert that we have 'the alternative'. Instead we have attempted to create a 'space' in which different perspectives on mental health and therapy can be developed and, crucially, where a different kind of relationship between professionals and users can begin to be established. We have engaged directly with the challenges derived from the writing of Foucault (and others) and the challenges presented by the emerging user movement, and sought to imagine how mental health work could be different.

I moved to Bradford in 1995 and, alongside Val Rhodes (the team manager) began to recruit a team of nurses, care assistants, social workers and others who wanted to work in home treatment and who shared a wish to reach beyond the concepts of traditional psychiatry. However, the first person employed was Peter Relton, an ex-user of mental health services in Bradford. Peter's job title is 'service user development worker' and his job description was initially somewhat vague. I shall discuss below the contribution he has made to the development of the team philosophy and its way of working. Medical support to the team is from a Clinical Medical Officer grade doctor (CMO; currently, a trained GP). I was initially employed as a part-time consultant with the team (3 days a week) but over time the need for my clinical involvement has lessened and I now work with other parts of the service besides home treatment.

The team offers 24-hour support to people in a mental health crisis who would otherwise be admitted to hospital. A shift system operates with two people always rostered to work from 1 p.m. until 9 p.m. These workers are then available on an on-call basis for the rest of the night. The other workers are present from 9 a.m to 5 p.m. The team works 7 days a week. Clients of the service are visited regularly in their place of residence. These visits are usually on a daily basis but can be as often as three times a day or as little as once or twice a week. Times of visits are negotiated with clients. Telephone contact is an important feature of the service and clients will often telephone at night for reassurance and support. If there is no telephone in the home a mobile phone is provided for the duration of the team's involvement.

Over time, a philosophy of care emerged which is now written down and available to clients and their carers, and to visitors to the service. This emphasises the importance of trust and acknowledges that traditional ways of working with people in distress have often served to render genuine trust untenable. Crucially, the philosophy commits the team to working with the client's own understanding of their problems. It states that although at times it may need to challenge some of the client's beliefs it will not seek to undermine their perspective on themselves or their world. The team philosophy states:

> The team recognises the importance of supporting individuals and helping them define and make sense of their own experiences in their terms, rather than

staff imposing their own definitions and labels. Staff will sometimes challenge the ideas of users but will not silence their ideas or undermine the confidence of the user. This involves staff being prepared to accept and work with ideas and beliefs that may differ from their own.

Over time, the home treatment team has begun to understand its encounters with clients in terms which, increasingly, owe little to traditional psychiatry. The diagnosis of schizophrenia is not used (see below) and other words from a psychiatric vocabulary are used tentatively. The idea that clients have 'symptoms of illness' is still present but other non-medical ways of understanding people's problems are also used. However, as the home treatment team works within the constraints of the statutory sector, it is not possible to shed all the functions of a traditional psychiatric service. Thus, for example, when the risks of caring for someone at home become too great there is an obligation on the team to consider the need for hospitalisation and some clients of home treatment eventually end up being detained. However, the team is committed to struggle, in whatever ways are open to it, to avoid this. In what follows, I shall attempt to outline some features of the service which demonstrate the desire to put principles into practice. I believe that these features reflect a genuine effort on the team's behalf to shed a reliance on the concepts of psychiatry and an attempt to move in a 'postpsychiatry' direction.

Service user involvement

From the outset it was thought crucial to involve a critical service user in the development of the service. The post of service user development worker was mentioned above. Peter's role has changed over time but essentially he has been focused on changing the culture of the team (Relton 1999). He attends all the clinical and business meetings and sometimes has direct involvement with clients of the service. However, the focus of his work has been developmental. He challenges ways of thinking and talking about clients and has forced team members to struggle against a sense of 'them and us' in relation to the understanding of clients' circumstances and needs. It is apparent that his perspective has gradually been internalised by other team members (including myself) and there are now different starting points for discussions about clients and their difficulties. Peter is now in charge of the training agenda for the service and, over time, strong links have been forged between team members and local user and survivor organisations. He also sits on most of the interview panels when the team is recruiting new workers.

Alongside the service user development post, local service users have also been involved with a steering group set up to advise on the evolution of the service. Initially only a couple of users were involved, but now, due to Peter's insistence, over 50% of this group are from service user backgrounds. The steering group helped draft the initial operational policy for the service and has guided its work over the years. In addition, the team wishes to recruit individuals who have had mental health service involvement to other roles apart from the specific developmental job. So far, one worker, who was previously a client of the service, has started to work in a health care assistant post. The team has shown a commitment to the involvement of service users in a meaningful way. It aims to be not simply a team of professionals but rather a group of individuals who come from different backgrounds and bring different perspectives and skills to their work. The goal is a situation where no particular perspective is privileged over others. Users of psychiatric services often have their criticisms of mental health care undermined when workers refer to a professional knowledge base which seems to justify questionable aspects of their practice. By systematically opening up the assumptions underlying psychiatric knowledge, postpsychiatry has the effect of 'levelling the playing field'. The home treatment service has sought, in practice, to establish a framework in which a more democratic form of user professional communication can take place.

The denial of psychiatric theories and frameworks

The service attempts to work with a 'needs led' approach and does not, for the most part, seek to diagnose the client's problems in a medical way. At times, a medical diagnosis is necessary and important, as when there is a suspicion that organic factors might be affecting the person's condition. The medical members have no compunction in arranging various medical tests if these are indicated and everyone who is admitted to the service has a medical examination by the CMO grade doctor. The point is that the team's interventions are not guided by psychiatric diagnoses and theories. Psychotropic drugs are used and occasionally the administration of medication does become a priority. However, these drugs are generally used on a symptomatic basis and not with the belief that they are curing a psychiatric 'disease' of some sort. Just as paracetamol sometimes relieves a headache brought on by worry and stress but does not eliminate the cause of the headache, so too it is our belief that some psychiatric drugs can offer a reduction in anguish and distress. However, we also believe that the benefits of these drugs have been exaggerated in the psychiatric literature and in the claims made by the pharmaceutical industry. (There is now an emerging mainstream literature which would question previous claims about the efficacy of antidepressant drugs; for example, see Moncrieff et al 1998. For an excellent discussion of the problems with antipsychotic drugs, see Thomas 1997, Chapter 6, 'A bitter pill'.) The home treatment team has attempted to limit substantially the amount of drugs being used, and there is evidence that this has been successful (Cohen 1999). Over 20% of clients actually reduce the amount of medication they are taking while on home treatment. In addition, echoing what was said in the last section, the home treatment team is concerned with the down side of psychiatric interventions and treatments and is particularly wary of the longer-term effects of these drugs.

Although it is virtually impossible to work in the area of mental health without using words from a psychiatric vocabulary, some words and labels carry a greater burden than others. Words such as 'depression', 'anxiety', 'manic' and 'paranoid' are sometimes used in team discussions in a descriptive way, but there is a particular concern to avoid invoking the concept of schizophrenia. This term is always more than a description of someone's state of mind; it is a diagnosis in itself and intrinsically invokes psychiatric classification and theory (Bracken and Thomas 1999). Many clients of the service have the experience of hearing voices. The team has looked to the theoretical and practical work developed by the Hearing Voices Network as an alternative to the psychiatric understanding which simply understands voices as morbid hallucinations (Romme and Escher 1993). One of the team members has produced a short booklet for clients outlining this perspective (Sheriff 1999).

Focus on engagement and negotiation

The home treatment team places a high priority on developing trusting relationships with clients of the service. With this in mind, 'engagement' and 'negotiation' are terms which are often heard at team discussions. There is a commitment to openness and honesty and in the initial sessions with a new client some effort is made to be clear what the service can and cannot do. Obviously engagement is not always possible and sometimes people who are referred to the service simply do not wish to be seen. A number of practical measures are in place to emphasise the importance of trust. For example, each client is asked if they would like to keep their own case notes during the period they are under the care of the service. Although there is nothing remarkable in this, and many medical services are experimenting with similar initiatives, for many clients this is an extremely important move. Users and their carers are encouraged to write their own entries in the notes and the ideal is a joint record of what has happened. It must be said that a majority of people do not take up the offer, but the team believes that it is important to make this a possibility. In effect, by offering client-held case notes, the team are saying: 'there is nothing that will be written about you that we would be unhappy for you to read'. This can be very reassuring. For some people who have had negative experiences with psychiatric services in the past the offer of keeping their own case notes can be a key factor which allows for engagement.

There is also an emphasis on negotiating care plans with clients and their carers. The team has sought to become skilled in complimentary therapies so that these can be offered alongside more conventional interventions. As discussed above, the focus of care is on practical considerations such as housing problems, benefit issues, employment and training, relationship difficulties and accessing leisure activities. Sometimes clients are assisted with cooking, or with trips out for shopping or to the swimming baths. Sometimes people just need someone to listen and to share what they are going through. Formal psychotherapy is rarely used. If relationships at home with relatives are at crisis point, a brief stay at a local hotel can be arranged. In addition, the team is piloting a 'home to home' scheme whereby clients of the service can be placed for a short period in the homes of members of the public who have been recruited. These 'hosts' are paid a fee and offer a safe bed, a meal and conversation in a non-institutional environment.

Efforts are made to avoid follow-up by the psychiatric services, if at all possible. Clients are encouraged, and helped, to access longer-term support through informal networks such as friends, church and religious communities and user organisations such as Mind in Bradford, one of the few user-controlled local Mind associations. Sometimes, longer-term practical support is arranged from social service funded agencies and housing association staff. If psychiatric service follow-up is required this is established through the local community mental health team and the outpatient clinic. The Care Programme Approach (CPA) is used if clients are in need of a key worker.

The priority of values

There is a great deal of interest at present in the concepts of 'clinical effectiveness' and 'evidence-based practice'. The essential idea at the heart of this emerging discourse is that science should guide clinical practice. It is proposed that substantial progress could be made in clinical practice if this was more focused on the research literature about the effectiveness of treatments and procedures. Psychiatry has taken up this agenda and many in the profession propose that the 'evidence-based practice' framework will be the answer to many of the discipline's current difficulties. From what has been written above it should come as no surprise that I am less than enthusiastic about this discourse. Although I am not against the idea of decisions being based upon evidence, I do believe that there are real problems in the way the current discourse is developing. To me this simply involves a restatement of the old Enlightenment project. Perhaps its emergence now, in the age of postmodernism and uncertainty, is akin to the emergence of various forms of religious fundamentalism which have appeared in the past 20 years. In the face of uncertainty and multiple realities, it is comforting to many to retreat to the arms of some set of fundamental truths, be these religious, philosophic or scientific.

The clinical effectiveness framework ignores the role of values in shaping research. My argument is that all of medical science and practice is premised on certain assumptions about the nature of the self and the world. However, nowhere is there more evidence that values are built into diagnostic categories than in the world of psychiatry. This becomes clear from the historical work of Foucault (discussed above), but has also been demonstrated through the work of a number of medical anthropologists (for a good overview of this work, see Gaines 1992). Even a cursory examination of psychiatric classifications reveals them as value laden. In the nineteenth century, American psychiatrists wrote treatises about the problem of drapeto-mania, a disease of black slaves, the main symptom of which was a tendency to run away (Fernando 1995). Up until 1973, homosexual-ity was included in classifications of disease (Bayer 1981). The diag-nosis of posttraumatic stress disorder was included in the DSM-III of 1980 after a long battle between various interest groups (Young 1995). The diagnosis of depression is loaded with values derived from western culture (Kleinman and Good 1985) and the concept of schizophrenia is predicated on a strong notion of the bounded self, again a concept not accepted by many peoples on the planet (Fernando 1988).

The home treatment team works in the centre of Bradford and its catchment area includes a large number of immigrant communities. Many of these communities have orientations and values different from those of the host community. The home treatment team is committed to respecting these different values and frameworks and seeks not to impose its own assumptions. The team has attempted to establish links with religious healers and voluntary sector support organisations from ethnic minority communities.

On a broader level, the home treatment team has sought to base its practice on values rather than on the theories or diagnoses of psychiatry. It could be said that, for the team, a concern with evidence-based practice is always secondary to value-based practice. Indeed, the former is actually dependent on the latter. What evidence is judged useful and acceptable will always be dependent on the orientation of the person making the judgements. For exam-ple, many people in the black community in Britain find the discourse about high levels of schizophrenia in their community (a discourse developed largely by academic psychiatrists) unacceptable because of the assumptions it makes (Sashidharan and Francis 1999).

In its work the home treatment team attempts to keep the issue of values to the fore. Instead of questions such as 'what is the diagno-sis?', the team asks 'what does this person need at this stage?', 'how can we help this person cope with this crisis without a loss of dignity?', 'how can we help this person avoid coercive interven-tions?'. While recognising the pain and suffering involved in states of madness the team attempts to avoid the assumption that everything to do with madness is negative.

Conclusion

The home treatment team has been operational for about 4 years. During this time it has operated in a large catchment area (70000 population) with high levels of deprivation and social dislocation. Although it has taken some time to integrate the service with other aspects of the mental health system in the city (Bracken and Cohen 1999), in the 12 months from July 1998 there was a dramatic decrease in bed occupancy (to under 50% of the occupancy level prior to the development of home treatment). It is clear that home treatment (operating with a different philosophy) is able to offer a practical alternative to hospitalisation for many people in crisis. As mentioned above, the team did not start out with a clear postpsychiatry framework. However, in my opinion, as time has gone on and they have struggled to develop an alternative service, their ideas and practice have begun to move in a postpsychiatry direction. This struggle has demanded a real commitment from the team members to reflect critically upon their own work but in spite of this (perhaps because of it) morale has been very high. This has been the case across all staff groups. User satisfaction with the service has been very high (Cohen 1999).

My position is close to that of Sashidharan who writes:

> . . . today few people doubt the legitimacy of the argument that our psychiatric institutions fall short of the earlier romantic notions that they provide a haven for the vulnerable or cure and care for those in need. Increasingly, psychiatric hospitals, along with their satellite agencies, are identified as coercive institutions mediating a form of social control for the most dispossessed in our society (Sashidharan 1999).

A new framework for mental health services demands new thinking about the nature of the care on offer, a critical examination of traditional psychiatric theory and practice, and a prominent role for users in shaping the new services. In my opinion, innovation in mental health work has too often been thought of in terms of new 'techniques', or new ways of organising services more 'efficiently'. Too little critical attention has been directed towards the assumptions and values of services and how these shape the care received by users of such services. The Bradford Home Treatment Service has engaged directly with these issues and has shown that it is possible to work in a different way, even within the constraints of statutory provision.

References

Bauman Z (1989) Modernity and the Holocaust. Cambridge: Polity Press.

Bauman Z (1993) Postmodern Ethics. Oxford: Blackwell.

Bayer R (1981) Homosexuality and American Psychiatry: the politics of diagnosis. New York: Basic Books.

Bracken P (1995) Beyond liberation: Michel Foucault and the notion of a critical psychiatry. Philosophy, Psychology and Psychiatry 2:1–13.

Bracken P, Cohen B (1999) Home treatment in Bradford. Psychiatric Bulletin 23:349–352.

Bracken P, Thomas P (1998) A new debate in mental health. Open Mind 89:17.

Bracken P, Thomas P (1999) Let's scrap schizophrenia. Open Mind 99:17.

Cohen B (1999) Evaluation of the Bradford Home Treatment Service: Final Report. Bradford: University of Bradford.

Fernando S (1988) Race and Culture in Psychiatry. London: Croom Helm.

Fernando S (1995) Social realities and mental health. In: Fernando S (ed) Mental Health in a Multi-ethnic Society: a multi-disciplinary handbook, p. 17. London: Routledge.

Foucault M (1967) Madness and Civilization: a history of insanity in the age of reason, transl Howard R. London: Tavistock.

Foucault M (1977) Discipline and Punish, transl Sheridan A. London: Allen Lane.

Gaines A (1992) Ethnopsychiatry: the cultural construction of psychiatries. In: Gaines A (ed) Ethnopsychiatry: the cultural construction of professional and folk psychiatries, pp. 3–49. Albany: State University of New York Press.

Goffman E (1991) Asylums. London: Penguin.

Gordon C (1990) Histoire de la Folie: an unknown book by Michel Foucault. History of the Human Sciences 3(1):3–26.

Hampson N (1968) The Enlightenment. An evaluation of its assumptions, attitudes and values. London: Penguin.

Harvey D (1989) The Condition of Postmodernity: an enquiry into the origins of cultural change. Oxford: Blackwell.

Ingleby D (1980) Critical Psychiatry. New York: Pantheon.

Jameson F (1991) Postmodernism, or the Cultural Logic of Late Capitalism. London: Verso.

Kleinman A, Good B (eds) (1985) Culture and Depression. Berkeley: University of California Press.

Marx K (1977) Theses on Feuerbach. In: Marx K, Engels F (1977) The German Ideology, ed Arthur CJ. London: Lawrence and Wishart.

Moncrieff J, Wessely S, Hardy R (1998) Meta-analysis of trials comparing antidepressants with active placebos. British Journal of Psychiatry 172:227–231.

Newman F, Holzman L (1997) The End of Knowing: a new developmental way of learning. London: Routledge.

Oaks D (1998) A new proposal to Congress may mean daily psychiatric drug deliveries to your doorstep. Dendron 41/42:4–7. (The journal Dendron is published by the Support Coalition International, which is based in Oregon, USA.)

Parker I (1998) Against postmodernism: psychology in cultural context. Theory and Psychology 8(5):601–627.

Porter R (1987) A Social History of Madness. Stories of the insane. London: Weidenfeld and Nicolson.

Relton P (1999) Being out in the NHS. Advocate 22–24 May.

Romme M, Escher S (1993) Accepting Voices. London: Mind.

Rose N (1989) Governing the Soul. London: Routledge.

Roth M, Kroll J (1986) The Reality of Mental Illness. Cambridge: Cambridge University Press.

Sainsbury Centre for Mental Health (1998) Acute Problems: a survey of the quality of care in acute psychiatric wards. London: Sainsbury Centre for Mental Health.

Sashidharan SP (1999) Alternatives to institutional psychiatry. In: Bhugra D, Bal V (eds) Ethnicity: An Agenda for Mental Health, p. 211. London: Gaskell.

Sashidharan SP, Francis E (1999) Racism in psychiatry necessitates reappraisal of general procedures and Eurocentric theories. British Medical Journal 319:254.

Sheriff L (1999) Hearing Voices. Bradford: Bradford Home Treatment Service (available on request).

Solomon RC (1988) Continental Philosophy since 1750. The rise and fall of the self. Oxford: Oxford University Press.

Thomas P (1997) The Dialectics of Schizophrenia. London: Free Association Books.

Young A (1995) The Harmony of Illusions. Inventing post-traumatic stress disorder. Princeton: Princeton University Press.

CHAPTER 8

Providing intensive home treatment: inter-agency and inter-professional issues

BRUCE M. Z. COHEN

Summary

This case study describes the formation and interactions of an IHT team in Bradford. The inter-professional and inter-agency issues which arose in the first 30 months of operation are explored. Despite conflict with other agencies the home treatment team was deemed to have successfully met its aims.

Given the many practical and strategic obstacles encountered in the development of new community operations like home treatment services, maybe it is unsurprising that there is little time set aside for planning how the new provision will fit with other parts of the local system. Though there is often some consideration at managerial level which may be reflected in operational policies, the day-to-day inter-actions of professionals working together can be an entirely different state of affairs. In this chapter it will be shown that ignoring issues such as different work strategies, protection of professional skills, and demarcation of responsibilities can lead not only to inter-professional and inter-agency conflict – and thus erosion of the quality of care provided – but also the possible altering or demise of the new service. This will be demonstrated with reference to a case study of the Bradford Home Treatment Service which was evaluated over a 3-year period.

Background

Ledwith et al (1997, p. ii) note that though there is a healthy and respectable literature on the management and workings of the NHS within the confines of the hospital system, less has been reported on the management of community services, and hardly anything on the management of inter-agency projects (e.g. health and social services partnerships). Where reports have been produced on inter-agency activities they often show a pronounced confusion in the roles and responsibilities of each service. For example, a recent report by the King's Fund London Commission (1997) found 'systematic' problems with inter-agency working causing possible fragmentation within the provided mental health service. Reports such as these have cited a number of reasons for such confusion, including differences in cultural ethos, a lack of communication, and different perceptions of the service between management and workers on the ground. Recommendations for future services have included the development of a shared philosophy for the project, a strengthening of team as opposed to individual working, and building stronger communication links between agencies as well as between management and ground workers (see, for example, Brown et al 1991, Heginbotham 1999, Norman and Peck 1999). These issues will be returned to later in this chapter with reference to the case study outlined.

Case study: the Bradford Home Treatment Service

Methodology

This case study was made possible by the author's employment as a research fellow to evaluate the introduction and development of a new home treatment service in one sector of the city of Bradford. The evaluation was structured to be both formative and summative. That is, to both study the development of the service and provide feedback, as well as assessing whether the programme was an efficient and effective alternative to hospitalisation at the conclusion of the evaluation period. Quantitative measures and outputs from the evaluation have been reported elsewhere (see Cohen 1997a,b, 1999a, Bracken and Cohen 1999); for this case study considerable weight is given to the qualitative information which was collected over the same period.

The development of the Bradford Home Treatment Service goes back to 1995, though it was not fully operational until February 1996. The research fellow was employed in March 1996 for a 30-month period. To assess inter-professional workings as well as the inter-agency development tied to the project, individual open interviews were carried out with all current members of the home treatment team. These took place May to June 1996 ($n = 18$), and then October to November 1996 ($n = 19$). Observations and note-taking of the team's activities were carried out through the evaluation period, but was most intensely investigated July to October 1996 when one day every week was spent at the home treatment offices. At the end of the evaluation period a final focus group was carried out of home treatment to assess the shape of the team, the service, and future expectations. Observation work led to attendance at meetings with other agencies involved in the local health care set-up (e.g. training days, the home treatment Advisory Group meetings, ward rounds, etc.). Eleven formal individual open interviews (and one focus group) were completed with identified key 'other agency' workers who worked closely with the service between September and December 1996. Additionally, a focus group with hospital staff and an open interview with a member of social services management were obtained at the end of the evaluation period.

Background to the development of service

The development of the Bradford Home Treatment Service arose mainly from the initiative of the local health trust's chief executive who established a policy of promoting community mental health services (which had been a long-term aim of the trust). It was proposed to develop a scheme similar to that found in North Birmingham (see Sashidharan and Smyth 1992), where staff provided intensive support to people in their own homes in an effort to prevent admissions to the acute wards of the local psychiatric hospital. The health trust's chief executive then negotiated with the purchaser chief executive for funds to match those provided by the trust from their own efficiency savings. Social services then agreed to commit the resources of a social worker and two Asian support workers to the proposed team. A working party was set up to conceptualise the project and move it towards the initial recruitment of core staff for the service. This group included sympathetic consultants from the local psychiatric hospital, social services and health management, and a number of local user organisations.

In a telling paragraph from Ledwith et al's research on inter-agency working for ethnic minorities within the same geographical area, they comment on this early period of development of the service and how it was perceived by the different mental health agencies:

> In the early stages of our research, there was widespread lack of knowledge of the details or even the purpose of the new [home treatment] service. Among those involved in the planning process, there were considerable differences of view as [to] whether the service would be provided simply for a short time, crisis intervention over weeks for clients or whether it would involve longer term support over months, as and when needed (1997, p. 96).

The researchers conclude by stating that the way in which the home treatment service developed (i.e. without widespread agreement) suggests evidence of the relative unimportance of formal planning procedures where there is a strong will for radical change.

Pre-operations

By the autumn of 1995 an administrator, a nursing manager and a consultant had been recruited for the new service with a remit to assemble a team of multi-agency professionals and organise training towards the start of operations of the service in 1996. In the months that followed, both the consultant and the nursing manager played significant roles in shaping the philosophy and working practices of the team. The consultant described his position as, firstly, 'critical psychiatry' and then, latterly, 'postpsychiatry' (see Bracken, Chapter 9, this volume, and Bracken and Thomas 1998). The nursing manager had worked on acute wards as well as in the community with a mental health team for the homeless. Like a number of the home treatment team, she had become quite disillusioned with health practices and saw the project as a way she could stay within nursing and change these practices. She commented on the new service,

> 'I think we should be working quite differently, so I think one of our objectives should be that we try and challenge what's been done and try and work differently, I think that's the thing that's most difficult to do. To not just reproduce what's at [the psychiatric hospital] in the community.'

Admirable notions, but could such a philosophy of alternative care be sold to a multi-agency team coming from different – often highly prescriptive – work cultures, and could a new service survive in this form in the face of the dominant health and social care system within which they worked?

Along with the three social services staff pledged to the team, 11 community psychiatric nurses were appointed (consisting of eight qualified and three unqualified members of staff, reflecting all the major grades from team leader to assistant community psychiatric nurse), one clinical medical officer (CMO), and a quarter-time community psychiatric nurse to specifically liaise with the local community mental health resource centre (CMHRC). Significantly, a service user development worker was also appointed to work 4 days a week with the team. Emphasis was placed on training from the start, with 3 weeks of intense induction for the purposes of team building, introduction to other statutory and voluntary sector organisations in the area, and discussion of the new service's Operational Policy and with it the aims, objectives and overarching philosophy of the project.

A draft Operational Policy for home treatment had been developed by the advisory group together with the appointed consultant and the nursing manager before the recruitment of the home treatment team. This document has been revised by the team a number of times since, but the main themes have not been radically altered. The Operational Policy (Bradford Home Treatment Service 1996) states that the team will work together in an egalitarian way, all members of the team should be encouraged to share their viewpoint with others, members should be respected for their skills, experiences and opinions, and there should be a move away from the hierarchical system used in nursing and a move towards the group as the decision-making body. Similarly the philosophy for working with users respects their point of view, and encourages staff to understand and work with users in distress. Alternatives to medication should be facilitated, and hospitalisation should be discouraged. Staff translated this broadly as a move towards a 'social model' of care and away from a 'medical model'. So the Operational Policy emphasised that home treatment should not only be an alternative to hospitalisation, but also offer an alternative model of care. This led some other local professionals to conclude that home treatment had set themselves up 'apart' and 'against' other parts of the local system. This issue will be discussed more later in the chapter.

The locums cometh: the first year

The first year is always going to be the hardest for a new team and it is to the credit of team members and other professionals involved that most realised this reality; the notes and interviews carried out are full of references to 'teething difficulties', 'finding their feet' and 'development issues'. Nevertheless it was evident that the cohesion and morale of the team could easily be affected during this period by changes in the wider infrastructure as well as internal perceptions of the team's performance.

The team started taking referrals in mid-February 1996. For the first few months work was slow; it was only by the summer that home treatment were getting near to filling their maximum number of 12 client places (in July 1996 there were only two admissions to the hospital from home treatment's sector, the lowest on record). Unfortunately it was at this time that the sympathetic consultant for the sector left the hospital. In her place came a succession of locum consultants who were unfamiliar with home treatment and felt it unsuitable in many cases. The reasons for this attitude from the locums can be summarised as a lack of knowledge of what the purpose of home treatment was (many saw it as an avenue for early discharge rather than as an alternative to hospital), and also a highly medicalised idea of what appropriate treatment for mental health users should consist of. Consequently, home treatment referrals declined whereas hospital admissions increased towards the end of 1996. An evaluation report of the first year of operations (see Cohen 1997a) showed that home treatment had reduced hospital admissions from the sector by 25% on the previous year and that the quality of the service was felt to be much better than hospital care by the users. However, the cost of service (per 'bed' day) was higher compared with the hospital. Reasons for this were summarised as due to low turnover of users on the service and the low number of spaces for users available on home treatment. Inappropriate admissions (i.e. not 'acute' or 'severe' cases) was also highlighted as a problem. This and other problems were tied closely to the arrival of the locums and the lack of control of the referral process the team had.

The fight-back: 6 months city-wide

Mindful of the home treatment service's need to be taken as a serious alternative to hospital and the damage the current situation could do for credibility locally, the service's consultant negotiated the expansion of the service from the one sector to all five in Bradford by January 1997, meaning that the service could take referrals from across the city. The maximum number of users the service would accept at one time was provisionally 15 but the total could get closer to 20 on some occasions. The expansion of the catchment area had the positive effect of seeing the number of users rapidly increase, and showing other consultants the usefulness of the service in redirecting users from hospital treatment. However, the staff became concerned by the amount of time spent in travelling across the city, and the impact this was having on their time with users. Working at an optimal level allowed the team to further assess the nature of the service, and how to maximise efficiency within team and inter-agency interactions.

Complete control? A further 12 months

By the summer of 1997 a new and sympathetic consultant had been employed by the trust to cover home treatment's original sector of operations. The service ceased its city-wide operations and went back to working mainly in this sector, additionally taking a limited number of referrals from a neighbouring sector where the hospital consultant was also very positive towards the service's input. Due to close working relationships between the home treatment and sector consultants, when users entered the psychiatric system at these points, preference was given to the home treatment service. An evaluation report produced after 12 months of these workings showed 81% (42) of users surveyed found home treatment 'better' or 'much better' than hospital overall, compared with only 12% (6) finding hospital 'better' or 'much better' than home treatment. Further interviews with users who had received hospital treatment only, found that less than half of those interviewed felt hospital had been a good experience for them (see Cohen 1999a, 1999b). The Bradford Home Treatment Service also resulted in a reduced number of users in hospital, and was found to be cost-effective (see Cohen 1999a).

A going concern: into 1999

Despite political manoeuvrings, a current re-sectorisation of the city, and a degree of staff turnover, the production of the final evaluation report together with the influence of key players and current government policy initiatives have helped to further secure the Bradford Home Treatment Service's place within the local community mental health care system. The service has been nominated for a number of national awards for good practice, and received a number of grants to further programme initiatives. With local re-sectorisation currently taking place, it looks likely that two further home treatment teams will be created within the Bradford area as a direct result of the success of the first project.

Inter-professional working

At this point we should remember that the home treatment team had to equip themselves for a variety of changes to their previous practices; most obviously this was the questioning of their interactions with mental health users on home treatment, but there are also other factors that workers had to take on board simultaneously. Given the team wished to change their way of working and generally challenge the medical philosophy of care traditionally taken with users, there were bound to be points of professional strain and angst at a change to their practices, and also periods of resistance to changes which were brought about. This discussion gives examples which illustrate the main barriers encountered to the successful inter-professional work of the home treatment team and any solutions witnessed that alleviated these tensions.

Training, evaluation and review

The initial 3 weeks of training before the start of operations was generally welcomed by staff as necessary and useful, especially for team building, but also for awareness and knowledge of the related public and voluntary sector organisations they would be working with in the future. However, the general view was that more time could have been devoted to discussing the philosophy of home treatment's work with clients, given it was stated in the Operational Policy that staff would be working differently with users (e.g. respecting users' views, resisting medication, challenging the dominant medical ethos, etc.). It seems clear that there was the potential in this lack of discussion to cause early tensions between team members who might have conflicting philosophies. Generally the feeling was that 2 weeks would have been adequate and that there was too much information to absorb at one time; 'we'd got to saturation point', stated one member of staff.

One thing that is relevant to our discussion here is that the home treatment service had adequate mechanisms to be able to deal with conflict and problems when they arose. At first there were too many meetings, which were generally too long and from which clear decisions were not often made. This is often cited as one of the problems of the team-as-decision-making-body which comes under criticism from others. However, some members of the group were able to identify and clarify the need for constant review of procedures and practices taking place at home treatment. There was also an emphasis on the need for away-day (or half-day) reviews as often as could be facilitated when required (bearing in mind the availability of members of staff and the need to cover the service at all times). An example of this efficiency is that by the time the research fellow had highlighted such 'teething issues' in a developmental report to home treatment (see Cohen 1997b), the team had already reviewed and altered practices for meetings, hand-overs, etc. The team also had another review specifically to discuss issues highlighted in this early report.

Different work cultures: the health–social work divide

As the dominant force within home treatment, the healthcare professionals imported many of their systems of operation such as the staff rota, the hand-over meeting and management forms such as the nursing care plan. This had the initial effect of isolating non-healthcare professionals on the team, with one nurse commenting at the time that, 'I genuinely feel that there is still a division between nursing staff and people who do nine-to-five because it's a different job.' The 'staff rota' included only nursing staff and demarcated time slots in terms of nursing shifts, which work on a 24-hour, 7-day-a-week cover basis, rather than a 9 a.m. to 5 p.m. daily rota as might be in place for other groups of workers. This had a knock-on effect in terms of case work with users. Nursing staff looked to other nursing staff to hand over to, which ensured that up-to-date information on the progression of care was maintained throughout the 'shifts', but served to further exclude non-nursing personnel from a fair share of case work with users. The health–social work divide was most clearly evident in early work patterns through the separation of roles. Social workers were called upon when 'socially related' issues arose for users on the service (e.g. applications for Disability Living Allowance or unemployment benefit, housing problems, social fund applications, child protection, etc.), but for the issues considered 'health orientated' such as medical interventions, one-to-one support, counselling, etc., nurses were assumed to be the appropriate professionals to oversee this care.

It was again through the system of home treatment internal review that the issue between nursing and non-nursing staff was highlighted and began to be dealt with. An amount of mutual understanding helped in bringing about more cohesion in the group, and this could be reinforced by different professionals demonstrating in their feedback from working with clients as to what they could offer in terms of 'care' and 'treatment' in the home setting. As one social worker on the team mentioned, she had not been treated as an equal to begin with,

'But now, after I've marketed my role in the team, no problem. The first time I went out to do an assessment someone said "are you all right to do that?!" I'm equally qualified, so it was quite quickly ironed out.'

Other methods of integration were also put in place after away-days had highlighted the problems of different working patterns. For example, all staff members were added to the team rota, and the team was encouraged to share out clients equally among all staff members and to work jointly on cases whenever this was possible and acceptable to the service users. Different members of staff were also encouraged to lead discussions on an aspect of their community health work at feedback meetings so as to facilitate understanding of different people's knowledge and skills base. (This was particularly useful in giving the service user development worker a platform with which to challenge the working practices of professionals at the service.)

The nursing hierarchy

Although home treatment was attempting to work in an egalitarian manner, rather than mirroring the strict grading system within nursing, it soon became clear that at least some of the nursing staff were turning back to their established 'professional roles' rather than challenging them. This was highlighted in some observed acts of staff members who were seen as 'junior staff' in spite of their increased responsibilities on home treatment. One nurse gave an example where she had been with a distressed client. She was telephoned by another member of home treatment to send some blood samples to the local hospital. She enquired if there was anybody else who could do this as she was with a client, but was told there was nobody else available. On returning to the home treatment offices she found four other people there who could have done this task, but was informed by one 'senior' member of the team that 'G grades don't do blood'. At the initial training it was said that the team would get away from this situation but it was still being used by some. As the majority of staff sided with the egalitarian working methods, and the roles of each member of staff became less demarcated over time, staff who tried to enforce the old system of nursing became marginalised. The general view was reflected by one nurse who stated,

> 'With this team, the roles are a lot more blurred . . . I come from a school of thought where an A grade can do what an F grade does as long as they know what they're doing and they're supervised, I'm happy with that . . . I accept the fact that people can be autonomous as long as we are aware that they are practising safely.'

Professional skills base

From the literature on professional knowledge and skills (for example, see Turner 1995), it is suggested that a professional body attempts to monopolise an area through promoting their own practices, qualifications and skills as the appropriate ones, while attempting to exclude and marginalise the skills and practices of others. With different professionals coming together within a group there were bound to be some points of tension as professional workers negotiate the boundaries of what they consider their areas of expertise. Further to this, though, tensions came into play when adapting a new theoretical and practical approach to user care that could in theory undermine the skills base of all the professions involved. One worker noted,

> 'Some people [were] being very protectionist about their own roles and responsibilities . . . And I just felt for most people there's been a slipping back into whatever ways they might have functioned before. It felt like people were trying to

live up to what we had set ourselves as a team for a while, but people end up feeling insecure about certain things and because of that, revert back to old ways of doing things . . . I suppose a lot of people are a lot less radical than they think they are in some ways, it's like they still operate within a system that is only going to allow you to go so far. And a lot of people do get insecure because they don't want to lose their job, it's that sort of climate.'

In later interviews, staff also noted their early anxieties at 'letting go' of their professional skills but also coming to an understanding of the ability of being in a team which allowed the creation of new skills. Coming up to 12 months of employment, one staff member reflected the feelings of many on the team when she said,

'I'm a lot more clear about working with clients. At first I thought I was simply losing the skills I had gained in my previous job, but now I'm working with clients, I've actually been gaining new skills and knowledge . . . That's the good thing about this job, it has flexibility for you to expand your role if you want – it's up to you.'

Inter-agency working

In spite of the involvement of other statutory and voluntary sector agencies in the setting up of the home treatment service and the continued dialogue with other professionals through the daily workings of the team, it has not always been plain sailing between home treatment and other parts of the local mental health system. Sometimes tensions appeared in the form of practical situations which occurred at the day-to-day level between home treatment workers and other professionals over issues such as supervision and working methods. On other occasions it was the general perception of the home treatment service's operations which appeared to challenge the work of other professionals. In this section we look at different parts of the local system and their relations with home treatment before offering some general issues that are raised by this discussion.

The psychiatric hospital

As the hospital consultant for home treatment's sector was the main gatekeeper for referrals to the service, it was essential that good lines of communication and working practices were maintained with this person and the hospital staff generally. Relations at first were positive, with some of the home treatment staff having worked on the ward previously and there being good contact with the consultant and the ward nursing manager. This situation began to change as a succession of locums began admitting more users to the ward rather than to home treatment. The nursing manager explained at the time,

> 'The main problem, that we're trying to deal with, is that our admission rate has gone up. Our consultant left in May and she wasn't replaced, we've had two locums . . . and the referrals weren't going to home-based treatment, people wouldn't refer even if the nurses asked them to. Duty doctors wouldn't listen to the ward nurses, people weren't being assessed, we've had 10 or 11 clients in for that area, which is the most we've ever had in months for that area.'

A change in the type of clients entering home treatment was noticeable, as one member of home treatment staff commented, 'we seem to be getting people who don't need that much intensive input and need to be referred on to something else, that's what I'm finding, we've had a few inappropriate referrals.' Later, when home treatment had gained control of the referral process for the sector, ward staff began to feel powerless when home treatment staff delivered what were seen as 'inappropriate clients' at the hospital door and 'dictating' treatment. When the locums were in charge of the referrals it appeared that home treatment staff were being disadvantaged; now the ward staff felt at the mercy of a system outside of their control. Ward staff were becoming frustrated by the attitude and power that home treatment staff now had. One ward nurse noted of home treatment that,

> 'Nine times out of ten [the home treatment team] just bring the patient on and say "they're for admission", they're not, they're there for assessment but obviously they're under the assumption that they're for admission. It does make it hard for us, because we have to accept these people, even though we know it's wrong, and that shouldn't be the case.'

Perceptions of home treatment's philosophy as 'antipsychiatric' and thus 'anti-hospital' added to this deteriorating situation. By the end of the evaluation period the ward staff were left feeling emasculated by the imposition of home treatment on their work. Hospital staff were not against home treatment's more socially orientated model of care, but could see that compared with home treatment, hospital is a place where 'I come on the ward and the nurses'll give me tablets and, you know, inject me . . . and that's it . . . whereas you know we do try and do more.' The ward staff felt deskilled by the expansion of such community services, as well as the segregation of activities within the hospital system, meaning that counselling, phys-iotherapy, etc., were now being undertaken by different hospital departments and specialists. One charge nurse stated that he would like his staff to be involved in similar types of care to home treatment on the ward, but that,

> 'Referring people out to specialists to give care [has made] our position redun-dant. You know we might as well be prison officers with keys and keep the door locked and refer people out to different specialists to give care and that's not how I see the job. We used to actually do it on the ward, all the activities, the relaxation groups, were all done by ward-based nurses on the ward . . . Just over the years, I don't say we've given away roles, it's just other departments have sprung up and taken our role off us.'

The resentment of home treatment by ward staff appears to be only part of the issue. The bigger issues concern under-resourcing of the wards, the deskilling of nurses on the ward and a self-perception that staff are being left behind by the new developments in commu-nity psychiatry.

The Community Mental Health Resource Centre

A member of the Community Mental Health Resource Centre (CMHRC) for the sector was employed to act as a formal link between the service and home treatment staff. Though there was physically only a few hundred yards between the two services, they remained miles apart in terms of their perceptions of each other. This post was discontinued, as it became a quite negative role for the nurse to perform, which consisted of 'passing complaints back and forward which ain't good. . . . Communication breakdowns and things like that . . . you can do that on an individual basis.' This CMHRC was particularly understaffed and under-resourced at the time, and the introduction of home treatment as another point of referral on to them was seen as creating additional work problems for the CPNs at the CMHRC, as they explained,

> 'With the caseloads that we've got, I know it sounds awful, but sometimes when someone's admitted to the ward it's like one less thing to worry about for a

while. You do keep tabs on them, you do go and see them on the ward. But when somebody's quite ill, you just don't have that extra responsibility that you might have when they're at home . . . So as less people are admitted to the ward and more go on to home treatment, there's no let up in your work. I suppose really we just feel more pressured and it's not recognised, and nobody ever says "there's a bit of extra help for you", or people see home treatment as a bit of extra help for us, and we don't see it as creating much space.'

Direct resentment was also felt at the amount of resources which had been allocated to the new service by health managers in comparison with the under-resourcing of the CMHRC:

'The amount of resources that were allocated to home treatment, they've got a high staffing level and a relatively low ratio to clients. . . . I think most of the staff feel, like I said, resentful of all the resources they've had, and perhaps the amount of time they can spend with clients.'

These issues were also inflamed somewhat by the perception – similar to the hospital staff – of home treatment as an 'antipsychi- atric' or 'anti-medical' form of care. There was a feeling of difference and separation of the two services, although it was believed that they were both involved in the same treatment, as one nurse at the CMHRC noted,

'I think [the home treatment staff] felt as though a lot of their aims were differ- ent to the rest of the service, but I think really we're all aiming, when you're working in the community, to keeping somebody at home . . . if they came round more to seeing that. I think we're bogeymen or something – you know we're very medical. But we're not, we use a lot of psychosocial interventions as well . . . There's a whole different language [between the CMHRC and home treatment]. . . and we're both doing the same thing.'

Generally the staff at the CMHRC wished for some recognition by home treatment and the health managers as to the amount of work they were undertaking given their lack of resources. The CPNs felt that, 'perhaps some acknowledgement of what we do would be nice, you know, you might feel more like reciprocating.' The home treatment staff also seemed aware of these issues, and it had a knock- on effect of keeping users on home treatment longer than was neces- sary as to try and help alleviate the resource constraints at the CMHRC. In common with hospital staff, the conflict between the CMHRC staff and the home treatment service appears to be only part of a wider resentment at the current state of the local health system. Home treatment being perceived as having an 'alternative' philosophy to working with users has only served to heighten this tension between the different services.

Social services

As social services were directly involved in the operations of home treatment, and had management representation on the service's Advisory Group, it might be assumed that better relations were nurtured between them and the home treatment service. Certainly the social services were less concerned with home treatment's change in the model of care, and welcomed a move towards more egalitarian ways of working together. However – similar to the concerns of some staff in the home treatment team – social service's concerns focused on the dominance of the medical and nursing staff, and the health system's operation in the team. One social services manager stated,

> 'I guess what I do have a concern about is the idea that [home treatment is] a joint health–social services operation and it isn't. I mean I think they're very fortunate that [the home treatment psychiatrist] is a 'non-medical' psychiatrist if you like, but I think staffing the team with primarily nurses, even if they're newly qualified, their training was medical, their training wasn't social . . . they come from a different background. And I wondered if it would have been more equitable to have more social workers in place as well.'

Different problems occurred for social services management and workers. Social workers outside the service felt that their many years of experience in dealing with clients were not being utilised, and that home treatment staff were sidelining them from the referral and case work process, allowing them only a secondary input. One local social worker complained that,

> 'When [the previous hospital psychiatrist] was the sector consultant, certainly with people I was working with, if I felt people needed to be in hospital, I would contact her, we'd talk about it and then they'd go into hospital, she didn't necessarily need to see them. When home treatment came online it was kind of like "[the consultant] has to refer", so it would be a case of me speaking to [the consultant], her saying yes home treatment would be OK, me getting back to home treatment saying this is the case.'

Working was better when a home treatment social worker was involved with the outside social workers, and between them they could negotiate issues and case work to mutual satisfaction, as another local social worker pointed out,

> 'Accessing the service can be difficult in terms of having a prescribed medical route, I've had headaches with people saying the duty psychiatrist definitely has to see somebody. . . And when you know somebody, and you think you can say where they've deteriorated to the stage where they need hospital. . . But there's others who will say "OK, we'll take the referral". . . That has been the case, but that's been social worker to social worker, I think it's easier for perhaps [the home treatment social worker] to kind of like side with my judgement really, because we come from similar backgrounds.'

Without this involvement social workers were finding the referral process that came into place with the introduction of home treatment harder to negotiate with, given that past work could be done less formally and with fewer people involved. Referral had become more bureaucratic and had led to additional barriers to successful working with users. Limited communication with the home treatment service appeared to leave the situation unresolved. At management level, professionals were also feeling sidelined after the initial process of setting up the home treatment service. It was felt that communication was only forthcoming from their social services staff on home treatment feeding information back to them, and through the irregular home treatment Advisory Group meetings. There was a feeling within the social services management that home treatment were making a lot of important decisions without any social services input, and this was felt partly due to social services being seen as a 'junior partner' in the new service because they provided only three of the staff for the team.

The home treatment service was developing but social services did not seem to be involved centrally in decisions or discussion on the direction of the service. The social services manager expanded on these themes, noting that,

> 'We are like satellites away from it . . . I think . . . with any new team there are some teething difficulties and that should be accepted. I think they're trying to run the services, but . . . they think it should be for people with long-term mental illness who can be seen at home, but there have been occasions where I

felt, was it being used more as a crisis service? . . . That is how I see it . . . If the policies have changed why don't I have the latest operational policies?'

As Ledwith et al (1997) outlined, different groups of workers had different perceptions of how the home treatment service would work. As has been stated earlier, it was sometimes necessary for home treatment to change for political reasons as much as for service development reasons. Increased partnerships between health and social services have not always increased understanding, and the perceived dominance of health management in the development of the home treatment service has obviously caused social services management some irritation. At the same time it was also noted in some of the research observations with home treatment staff that the team could become equally irritated with the social services management when joint meetings were held on development issues. It was often felt that social services were unlikely to act positively to innovations suggested by the team for the development of the service, and in their own way social services appeared over-bureaucratic to these health professionals.

The voluntary sector

In contrast, links with voluntary sector organisations seemed to work well from both points of view. These links were particularly nurtured between home treatment staff (especially the service user development worker) and the user organisations and support groups who offered a variety of activities which users could be directed to. User organisations appeared particularly encouraged by home treatment's working methods and their use of these organisations, with the manager of one group commenting that,

'What I've found is that [the home treatment staff have] referred a lot of clients to us which is good for us, and shows that they're thinking about what we do: support people out of hospital and to realise people's needs that they might need an advocate, which I think is quite positive. . . At least the home treatment team are giving us this recognition and I think it's a step forward. Like going up to hospital and going on the wards, you get a good response sometimes, sometimes it's lukewarm, other times they just look at you as if you've just crawled out of the woodwork – they probably think "those stupid advocacy people again!".'

Good links with local and national user groups were maintained through the service user development worker, and a number of voluntary sector members were also present on the service's Advisory Group. It seems interesting that home treatment had better relations with groups closer to the users than with other professional groups.

Discussion

Ramon (1996, p. 166) notes of multi-agency working that,

> 'The level of competition for power increases as the representatives of the different disciplines have a more equal say, but they may also wish to secure/increase the power of their own discipline. Alternatively disciplinary boundaries may become less important than they were before, and the internal team becomes the core of cohesion and identity for its members. This usually takes place where traditional forms of professional practice are open to critical discussion.'

Happily for the Bradford Home Treatment Service, the team has moved from the former to the latter position through the facilitation of critical discussion of mental health work. However, the local system of mental health as a whole fails to reflect the service's own ability to work together on a new basis, and the existence of home treatment has appeared to add to the lack of harmony between different organisations who are supposed to be working together on community health issues. This section discusses some of the ongoing difficulties of inter-professional and inter-agency working.

Communication

Communication was raised as a major issue by professionals in other agencies. For example, it was often stated that other professionals were unsure of exactly what sort of service home treatment was. Even if people did understand the general concept of home treatment, this was undermined by home treatment changing their own practices as the situations outlined previously called for the expansion of the sectors worked in, or the type of input which was possible with clients. One professional stated that,

> 'What I understood was that when [the home treatment service] started up, the philosophy was to prevent admissions to hospital, provide a service in the home.

> From what I've picked up recently . . . it's been more that they've intervened in
> that, and then they're given more work to follow-up and my understanding of
> crisis-management, from jobs I've had in the past, is that when the crisis is over,
> you pull out. They seem to be creating some needs which I'm not sure I would
> necessarily do if I was working in that way.'

It was also felt by other agencies that home treatment had 'high expectations' of what other agencies could do and how quickly these things should happen. At the same time home treatment staff have also been concerned about how to network and clearly communicate issues with their partner agencies, and have not appeared slow to try and deal with this problem. Talks, dissemination and feedback to other professionals has remained an ongoing process (this has included local feedback by the research fellow and dissemination of the evaluation results), but the situation has not particularly improved. The research continued to show that professionals often did not know what home treatment was there for. It appears that all sets of professionals are responsible for this liaison and to some extent the blame cannot be said to entirely lie at home treatment's door. There appear to be larger issues of how the local systems of health care communicate with each other, particularly at the management level of operation.

Management and grass-roots workers

Members of local health management tended to be very enthusiastic about the home treatment service, to the point of comparison with other parts of the system which were seen as less dynamic. As one senior health manager commented, the home treatment team were,

> 'An energetic group of vibrant people. Who, unlike some of their colleagues,
> have great enthusiasm, who are working far more flexibly than any other
> mental health staff in the Trust. . . I think it's far more difficult to work in a
> patient's home than on the ward.'

However, we have noted that there appears to be a difference in perception between what managers think is happening with services and what grass-roots workers are experiencing. This has been evident from the outset of the home treatment service, where the will of management has seen the service to operation without strategic planning necessarily keeping pace with the developments on the ground. Heginbotham (1999) has seen this as one of a number of 'splits' which is blocking multi-agency collaboration, and in turn breeds mistrust in management to understand and facilitate operational workings (see also Norman and Peck 1999).

Differing treatment philosophies

Challenging the traditional medical model of care, as well as changing the working practices within the home treatment team, has created a myth among other local professionals that the team is operating as 'outsiders' within an 'antipsychiatric' framework. This has probably strained relations further than they might otherwise have been, given that the introduction of a new service is always likely to be perceived as an initial threat to current systems of practice already in place. One local mental health manager pointed out some general problems of introducing a new service to an already under-resourced system of care:

> 'Initially I think there was a lot of apprehension anyway around certain areas of the Trust . . . people saying "I hear [the home treatment service is] into antipsychiatry", sort of shades of R. D. Laing, they weren't quite aware of what this new creature was going to be. . . On the one hand maybe it was threatening to certain people, on the other hand perhaps they were trying to fend it off by almost making it look different.'

The introduction of home treatment, with the necessary close monitoring and evaluation of the new provision, appears to have highlighted gaps in what was an already shaky system of local mental health care, where acute beds were in very short supply, the local CMHRC was overstretched, and generally networks of communication and cooperation between the health, social and community services were already poor (see Ledwith et al 1997). This current state of affairs in itself can be seen as reflecting wider national trends and should not be seen as particularly a home treatment or local issue alone. Nevertheless this issues remains a chief concern for the process of setting up alternative treatments in the community in the future. Conflicts and disagreements over professional ethos and ways of working together appear to form a smoke screen which hides the wider conflicts over resource allocations and successful strategies for the care and treatment of mental health users in the community.

Social services feel dominated by the power of the health services, user organisations still feel largely ignored (despite the growth of the voluntary sector more generally), hospitals feel under threat from community services, the community services in turn are themselves fighting over resources. Local conflicts and insecurities are reflected at a national level by the uncertainty of governmental policy on mental health care. One could argue – as local managers have – that given such a climate, the introduction of a new service was bound to cause inter-professional and inter-agency unrest. Granted that home treatment and local management could always have done more to overcome the obstacles that have since arisen for the new service in Bradford, it could also be claimed that – so long as the service had the ear of senior management – they did well to ignore or minimalise many of the external problems and focus on what best met the needs of local users. For all these potential obstacles and conflicts within the local health and social systems of operation, the Bradford Home Treatment Service has proved to be a success both in its approach to care of users with severe or acute mental health problems, and in its coherent approach to tackling team cohesion and development.

Conclusions

In terms of inter-agency working, the Bradford case study has high-lighted similar issues to other studies within the area:

- the general low morale of professionals working within commu-nity care and the mental health system generally
- a strong allegiance to uni-professional cultures
- the absence of a strong and shared philosophy of community mental health services
- mistrust of management solutions to the problems of inter-agency working (see Norman and Peck 1999).

In common with other commentators, the research has also high-lighted the fractured nature of current local community health care. Much can be blamed on previous legislation which has insisted on working together without any 'selling' to professional groups that this might be a good idea. Complaints around resources and planning operations appeared throughout this case study, and this is reflected in the Bradford Home Treatment Service by the difference in numbers of staff from the health service and the numbers from social services. However, what has also been highlighted by this case study is that the introduction of a new service into the local community healthcare system can manage to survive even within the present climate. The Bradford Home Treatment Service has appeared to succeed by placing itself 'outside' the dominant ethos of care and introducing an alternative set of professional values which can incorporate social service, health service and user/survivor philosophies. Consensus has come through the abandonment of the old lines of demarcation and professional values and, in turn, producing a new set of beliefs that allow for the incorporation of previous professional skills as well as the acquirement of new roles through placing the user of the service much more at the centre of the care regime.

Plenty of 'professional-bashing' goes on in the sphere of mental health at present. This chapter is not an attempt to add to this trend. Hopefully, the case study of home treatment in Bradford shows how inter-professional working can succeed despite less than perfect conditions. However, it must also be pointed out that the cohesion of the team was partially at the expense of the staff's previous professional skills base, suggesting that substantial relearning and retraining is necessary before different groups of professionals can come together in an effective way. The general failure of agencies to work together in Bradford reflects wider trends which block the often talked about 'seamless system of care'. As mentioned at the start of this chapter, given various constraints, the issues of inter-professional and inter-agency working appears comparatively low on the list of priorities for strategic planning and resourcing within mental health. As long as this continues to be the case, new projects such as home treatment services will continue to be sensitive to changes in local policy which may inhibit the teams establishing themselves as permanent entities. At the same time it is hoped that this chapter will help other projects achieve firmer foundations from which to progress in the future.

Acknowledgement

My thanks to David Cohen of Essex Social Services, with whom I had helpful early discussions about this chapter.

References

Bracken P, Cohen BMZ (1999) Home treatment in Bradford. Psychiatric Bulletin 23:349–352.

Bracken P, Thomas P (1998) A new debate in mental health. Open Mind 89:17.

Bradford Home Treatment Service (1996) Operational Policy. Bradford: Bradford Community Health NHS Trust.

Brown S, Cohen BMZ, Heald M (1991) Health Work in Hartlepool: Experiences of Providing and Receiving Mental Health Services. Middlesbrough: Teesside Polytechnic Centre for Local Research.

Cohen BMZ (1997a) Evaluation of the Bradford Home Treatment Service: Interim Report. Bradford: University of Bradford.

Cohen BMZ (1997b) Evaluation of the Bradford Home Treatment Service: Interim Report for Home Treatment Staff Development. Bradford: University of Bradford.

Cohen BMZ (1999a) Evaluation of the Bradford Home Treatment Service: Final Report. Bradford: University of Bradford.

Cohen BMZ (1999b) Psychiatric User Narratives. Bradford: University of Bradford.

Heginbotham C (1999) The psychodynamics of mental health care. Journal of Mental Health 8(3):253–260.

King's Fund London Commission (1997) Transforming Health in London. London: King's Fund.

Ledwith F, Husband C, Karmani A (1997) Promoting Inter-Agency Mental Health Provision for Ethnic Minorities. Bradford: University of Bradford Ethnicity & Social Policy Research Unit.

Norman IJ, Peck E (1999) Working Together in Adult Community Mental Health Services: An inter-professional dialogue. Journal of Mental Health 8(3):217–230.

Ramon S (1996) Mental Health in Europe: Ends, Beginnings and Rediscoveries. London: Macmillan.

Sashidharan SP, Smyth M (1992) Evaluation of Home Treatment in Ladywood: Results from the first two years. Birmingham: Birmingham Home Treatment Service.

Turner BS (1995) Medical Power and Social Knowledge (second edition). London: Sage.

CHAPTER 9

Developing intensive home treatment services: problems and issues

NEIL BRIMBLECOMBE

Summary

The evidence concerning IHT as an alternative to admission is summarised. Problems with an emphasis on inpatient care are discussed. Issues concerning the philosophy, structure, referral criteria and training needs of home treatment services are considered.

Introduction

Home treatment services providing an alternative to hospital admission potentially:

- increase choice for service users
- reduce the stigma and trauma frequently experienced due to hospital admission
- allow the resource of inpatient beds to be more available to those most in need of very high levels of supervision
- provide the opportunity for individuals to develop coping skills in their home environment.

This chapter briefly reviews the research evidence concerning home treatment services, and then considers a range of practical and philosophical considerations which affect the development and effectiveness of future home treatment services.

The argument for intensive home treatment services

There exists a substantial body of research evidence concerning home treatment services as an alternative to hospital admission. This has been accrued through controlled studies carried out over a period of more than 30 years. Results, even after taking difficulties in research design into account (see Orme and Cohen, Chapter 3, this volume), demonstrate that the majority of individuals with severe, acute mental health problems can be cared for by community-focused services with at least as good social and symptomatic outcomes as when cared for by services with a hospital focus (Pasamanick et al 1967, Langsley et al 1971, Stein and Test 1980, Fenton et al 1982, Hoult et al 1983, Marks et al 1994).

Those who purport to represent service users are persistent in their calls for the availability of crisis services and alternatives to admission (e.g. Richardson 1989, Wood 1994) and evidence demonstrates that where such alternatives exist these are valued equally or more highly than hospital admission by the majority of clients (Hoult, Rosen and Reynolds 1984, Marks et al 1994, Coleman et al 1998, Minghella et al 1998, Cohen 1999). Carers equally tend to prefer home treatment, although differences may not be noticeable in short-term involvement of services (Marks et al 1994). Home treatment services have been found to be cheaper than, or similar in cost to, more traditional services (Minghella et al 1998, Joy, Adams and Rice 1999, McCrone, Chisholm and Bould 1999).

The changing face of home treatment

Although the earlier research showed considerable advantages in symptomatic and social outcomes for community over hospital treatment, these differences have become less over time (Dedman 1993), presumably as even the most undeveloped services now have greater community resources. In the UK, for example, there has been considerable growth in community mental health centres (Sayce et al 1991) and the numbers of clients seen by community mental health nurses continue to increase (DoH 1999a). These resources, however, remain of limited value in meeting the needs of acutely ill clients, with the majority still operating only in office hours.

Many of the early home treatment services provided both acute community-based care, as an alternative to hospital admission, as well as longer-term 'assertive' follow-up. More recently there has been an increase in the number of acute services focusing on short-term interventions (see Orme, Chapter 2, this volume), able to respond rapidly to referrals from whatever sources are accepted within their own areas. Follow-up care is typically provided by generic community mental health teams or sometimes assertive community treatment teams.

Acute community services have also shown themselves able to offer a realistic alternative to inpatient admission for substantial numbers of individuals otherwise requiring hospital admission (Whittle and Mitchell 1997, Bracken and Cohen 1999, Brimblecombe and O'Sullivan 1999, Harrison et al 1999), are more acceptable to clients than standard hospital and community care (Cohen 1999), seem as effective in reducing symptomatology, and appear to be cheaper (Minghella et al 1998). In some cases IHT services have supplanted earlier attempts at providing alternatives to hospital, such as an acute day hospital (Creed et al 1991, Harrison et al 1999), proving themselves to be more effective still, in terms of preventing hospital admissions.

Suitability for home treatment

There is little UK-based research in relation to factors that determine admission to hospital for those with acute mental health problems (Smyth and Hoult 2000). There is also very little information concerning which individual characteristics are best suited to home treatment as opposed to hospital treatment and vice versa. Further research in this area is clearly required, as such information is vital in planning services and auditing their effect once established.

Limited evidence has suggested that individuals with personality disorder may be less likely to be successfully treated by home treatment services than those with other diagnoses (Bracken and Cohen 1999, Brimblecombe and O'Sullivan 1999). Individuals with suicidal ideation are often admitted to inpatient units by home treatment services, but the majority can still be treated in their own homes without this recourse (Harrison et al 1999, Brimblecombe 2000). Those with a previous history of psychiatric ward admission may be more likely to be admitted than others from home treatment (Dean and Gadd 1990).

Although all home treatment services appear to admit a proportion of clients after they have been taken on for home treatment, there has been considerable variation in evaluations of why these admissions take place and how frequently (Dean and Gadd 1990, Smyth and Bracken 1994, Minghella et al 1998, Brimblecombe and O'Sullivan 1999, Bracken and Cohen 1999). This remains another important area for further investigation.

Home treatment and older people

One area which has been particularly neglected in terms of research is that of home treatment as an alternative to admission for older people. Despite the recent increase in the numbers of crisis and IHT services, such services for older people with functional illnesses are rare (Mountain 1998).

Even when general reviews consider the structure and resources required to provide good services for older people, intensive home treatment appears to be left out of consideration (Spencer and Jolley 1999, Audit Commission 2000). No clinical rationale has been put forward to justify this division. The little that exists in the way of evaluation of crisis or home treatment services for this group suggests that such services may be of value. Ratna (1982) described a crisis intervention service for the over-65s with organic and functional problems, which appeared to reduce admission rates. Williams et al (1997) provided case vignettes to illustrate the work of a small team of four nurses providing IHT in Swansea, largely with the aim of providing an alternative to admission. The authors concluded that they had found that the team was especially effective in working with clients with major depressive disorders and paranoid states, as opposed to mild dementia, which was the area the team originally worked in. No statistics were given to support their conclusions. They described a range of interventions with clients, including providing and monitoring medication, assisting with bathing and diet, and supporting carers. Thompson (1999) provided a brief evaluation of a London home treatment service for clients with either organic or functional problems, which again appeared to reduce hospital admissions.

This limited number of studies is in spite of concern about how best to meet the needs of an expanding elderly population and the general shift from hospital-based to community-based services. It seems likely that older people would generally value the chance to stay in their own homes rather than enter hospital (Ellis 2000). Although there may be a greater likelihood of having to meet social and physical care needs in providing home treatment to an older age group, problems arising should not be insurmountable with adequate medical assessment and good liaison with, and responsiveness from, social care agencies. The introduction of the Health Act (HMSO 1999a) provides an opportunity for greater integration between health and social services, and should facilitate such joint working.

Problems with inpatient care

There is clear and persistent evidence of extreme pressure on acute inpatient psychiatric beds in many areas of the country (Hollander et al 1990, Hollander and Slater 1994). Such problems seem to constitute a rallying cry for those wanting more acute beds. However, we can rightly ask why, when it is evident that significant numbers of clients currently admitted could be cared for at home, given adequate acute community services. Where admission is necessary, problems in discharge are often related to lack of appropriate accommodation (Flannigan et al 1984, Fulop et al 1996) or lack of adequate care on returning home (Moore and Wolf 1999). Increasing the availability of acute beds rather than tackling the more general issue of lack of accommodation and adequate after-care services is, to say the least, missing the point.

Furthermore, there is evidence that for many clients admitted to inpatient areas the experience is far from satisfactory. Problems of boredom, little attention being given to social care needs, lack of privacy and clients (especially women) feeling threatened are all common experiences (Sainsbury Centre 1998). Claims have even been made that, for some individuals admitted when acutely psychotic, the experience of admission may be so distressing that, subsequently, symptoms are experienced meeting criteria for post-traumatic stress disorder (McGorry et al 1991).

Admission to wards may not only be unpleasant, but also unnecessary. Elwood (1999) found that 25% of admissions to an acute unit were considered 'inappropriate' by the very same junior doctors who carried out the admission! Studies of admissions show high rates of admissions (up to 52%) where the admitting doctor felt that had there been a suitable alternative available then admission could have been prevented (Flannigan et al 1984, Beck et al 1997).

However, it is apparent that IHT is often not even considered by many psychiatric professionals when thinking of suitable alternatives to hospital admission (Flannigan et al 1984, Fulop et al 1996). Providing a bed in a hostel, or day hospital care, tend to be those alternatives suggested by clinicians when asked. Anyone attempting to establish a new IHT service is likely to have to overcome the fact that previous experience, or lack of experience, of home treatment services may narrow the perceptions of what constitutes an alternative. Essentially, for many clinicians, direct exposure to the benefits of home treatment services may be needed before they see it as a real alternative.

Effects on beds

Although reduction in bed usage is commonly used as a prime measure of the 'success' of home treatment teams, the value of this measure can be ambiguous. The majority of studies, indeed, show marked reductions in bed usage in areas where home treatment teams are established (Dean and Gadd 1990, Marks et al 1994, Whittle and Mitchell 1997, Minghella et al 1998, Bracken and Cohen 1999). However, in a few cases bed occupancy has not significantly dropped. Interestingly, this seems to occur in areas which, at other times, have actually been able to show reductions (Audini et al 1994, Kwakwa 1995). This may be due to the number of admissions being successfully reduced, but with a consequence that pressure is reduced on inpatient medical staff to discharge early, because of no influx of new admissions. They are therefore able to keep other patients on the wards for longer periods. Is this a good or a bad thing? It is difficult to know without specific clinical reviews of those patients affected in this way. A further influence on length of stay may arise from the fact that those clients requiring admission where home treatment is available are likely to be those who are more difficult to treat and are likely to remain in hospital longer (Harrison et al 1999).

A factor directly related to the ability of home treatment teams to reduce bed occupancy – a goal of most services – is that of control of discharges. Evidence exists that, to make the maximum effect in this area, teams need to be able to control discharges as well as admissions (Audini et al 1994, Stephens and Huws 1997). The Southwark Daily Living Programme's experience of the effect of a loss of control over ward discharges and a consequent return to previous lengthy admissions (Marks et al 1994) illustrates the tendency of many psychiatrists to move away from truly community-based care, given an opportunity.

The limitations of home treatment services

Despite the largely positive evaluations of home treatment as an alternative to hospital admission, it is also apparent that it is no panacea. Even in areas with the most comprehensive community mental health services, some individuals with severe mental health problems will always require admission. Some will kill themselves (Cohen et al 1990). Improvement is no quicker in home treatment clients (Holloway 1995); many individuals will make only partial recoveries and require ongoing care (Stein and Test 1980). An effective home treatment service may also produce 'knock on' effects for inpatient services which present further challenges for already strained areas, for example by increasing the proportion of inpatients presenting with socially unacceptable or 'attention seeking' behaviour (Harrison et al 1999).

It is also apparent that higher levels of input from community staff, or smaller caseloads, do not on their own guarantee improved client outcomes (Muijen et al 1994). In fact, too much input from mental health services may even be detrimental to all those except the most needy (Wykes et al 1998). What seems to be important is the targeting of additional care (e.g. at the point where admission would otherwise be required) and by looking more closely at the interventions made by workers in terms of efficacy and appropriateness.

Although, arguably, most individuals with social stressors are best treated in an area where they can learn more effective ways of coping with such problems, undoubtedly a few will need and/or prefer a period of respite or asylum (although not necessarily in a hospital). Although, by and large, clients prefer home-based to hospital-based treatment, it is important that providers of home treatment services are not blasé about this. In particular, the exceptions to those satisfied with home treatment should be noted.

Clients do at times prefer hospital, and, in a significant number of cases, this is quoted as a reason that admissions take place rather than due to a particular need for inpatient care as perceived by home treatment team staff (Brimblecombe and O'Sullivan 1999, Cohen 1999). In reality this may be more accurately portrayed as the client's refusal to work with the home treatment team. Why should this be so? Some clients may see the positive elements of hospital, such as 24-hour care, company, accommodation and food, as more important than any negative aspect of hospital (Godfrey 1996). Therefore home treatment services need to address these issues, as far as possible, in negotiating an individual's care, and having access to other relevant services which can help in these regards.

Whom should home treatment services be for?

There is a possibility that the availability of responsive home treatment/crisis services may lead to a process of increasing the overall workload of psychiatric services, especially among those who 'formerly neglected their emotional problems' (Gerson and Bassuk 1980). Availability may increase the number of contacts with individuals who do not represent 'true' psychiatric emergencies, but, rather, use emergency services as a source of support. Whether this is a 'good' or 'bad' outcome is, of course, dependent on your point of view and on the criteria being used to evaluate a particular service. For example, Kwakwa (1995) is critical of an IHT team for seemingly taking on a new client group, as opposed to meeting the needs of existing clients who were more likely to have required hospital admission.

Although analysis of who is seen by a particular service is essential, caution is required when using variables such as diagnoses as a measure of the severity of individuals' problems. For example, the presence of psychosis increases the risk of suicide, but most people who take their own lives are not psychotic. Also, it is plain that those individuals admitted to hospital will be different in some way from those who can be treated at home. Any study which attempts to find that the same clients are being treated on the ward as at home should expect to find that this will not be the case. As previously mentioned, little work is yet available to begin to accurately distinguish which characteristics of an individual – symptomatic, behavioural, social and historical – will predict which type of service best meet their needs.

The issue of eligibility criteria would seem to be central to the practice of IHT. Seeing as few 'inappropriate' referrals as possible must be a priority for such a service, i.e. only seeing those who meet inclusion criteria, whatever those criteria might be. Again, Kwakwa (1995) describes the way in which the community team she examined spent so much time doing assessments that there was little time left for the process of home treatment. Clearly an acute community service with finite resources cannot be responsible for carrying out assessments on all referrals to mental health services, regardless of perceived urgency or treatment need. Nor can such a service 'take on' clients without careful consideration as to the severity and urgency of their need, as there are enormous numbers of individuals who may be seen by referrers as potentially benefiting from intensive treatment. All home treatment services who have reported their 'take on' rates following assessment show that some do not receive home treatment because they are in some way 'too severe', and require admission, whereas others are 'not severe enough', normally described in terms of not requiring an alternative to admission (Brimblecombe and O'Sullivan 1999, Harrison et al 1999). This applies whether referrals are accepted only from psychiatric services or from more open referral systems.

Even when eligibility criteria are apparently clearly stated, problems may still arise. A policy may state that there is a need for evidence, at the point of referral, which suggests the presence of an acute mental health problem potentially severe enough to warrant hospital admission. Yet even this is a vague concept. There are marked differences in different areas and between different professionals as to what constitutes a good reason to admit to hospital (Flannigan et al 1984). Mental health professionals generally agree that there is a need to avoid unnecessary admissions, but they seem to rarely agree on what constitutes 'unnecessary'.

Philosophies of home treatment

The question of whom home treatment services should be for raises the entire issue of the importance of the philosophy behind the aims of home treatment services. Are they there to provide the client with alternatives, or should the focus be on protecting NHS resources regardless of the client's preference? Most services appear to adopt the stance that the only 'alternative' being offered to the client is that of not being in hospital whenever this is possible. When admission takes place despite home treatment being the preferred option of staff, this is normally due to the fact that offering home treatment against the client's will is simply impractical (and may encourage 'acting out'), rather than it being simply down to giving the client a choice. Although this approach may be the only realistic and professionally responsible attitude to take, it should be borne in mind that much of the argument for the existence of home treatment services is that it is what clients want.

The Madison model of care (Stein and Test 1980) has been enormously influential in the development of home treatment services in the UK. The originators placed a high emphasis on the value of social care and expressed their belief that coping skills are best learned in the community. However, few pioneers in home treatment in this country appeared to take a clear philosophical stance on the meaning or ideals of home treatment. More recently others have explored such issues (Bracken, Chapter 7, this volume; Sashidharan 1999), arguing that home treatment services should challenge conventional psychiatric views of mental health problems and distress, and try to address the power imbalance between service user and professional.

The majority of services, who take no clear stance on such issues, cannot be seen as neutral in any debate. By not taking a clear position they are effectively accepting the status quo of psychiatry as it stands today. As new services continue to develop there is a need for philosophies to be carefully considered, as these will, in turn, influence both aims and practices.

Government policy

The DoH's position has at times seemed ambiguous in relation to community-focused care. In *Modernising Mental Health. Safe, Sound and*

Supportive (DoH 1998) the Government argued that 'community care has failed', although acknowledging that for many it had not. In fact, there is a distinct lack of evidence to support the idea that the general policy of shifting care towards a community-oriented model has 'failed' (Burns and Priebe 1999). When care is properly planned and resourced, community care for former long-stay patients is beneficial for most (Trieman, Leff and Glover 1999). There is no substantial evidence that a move towards shorter admissions is detrimental in itself (Johnstone and Zolese 1999). There is also good evidence that the most striking criticism of 'community care', that dangerous mental patients are increasingly killing members of the public, is simply untrue, with an average annual decline of 3% in the mentally ill's contribution to homicide statistics over the last 38 years (Taylor and Gunn 1999).

The Department of Health has cited a need for more beds, yet the inappropriateness of many admissions is acknowledged (DoH 1998). The Department has simultaneously identified a need to increase the numbers of 24-hour 'crisis' services, and the North Birmingham Psychiatric Emergency Team (typical in structure of many of the new home treatment services) is cited as an example of good practice. More recently, the National Service Framework (DoH 1999b) has asserted the need for 24-hour emergency assessment, yet without this being defined. The NHS Plan (DoH 2000) is more specific, calling for 335 'Crisis resolution' teams to be created over the next few years. Presumably many of these services will combine crisis assessment with home treatment functions. At the local level, among health authorities and trusts, there also now appears to be general agreement on the potential value of expanding the number of services providing home treatment (Owen, Sashidharan and Edwards 2000).

What enables successful home treatment?

Besides a political climate which allows for the development of more home treatment services, a variety of other factors are required to enable successful home treatment. These became evident even in the early days of developing community care in the UK. In 1958, a community-focused project in Worthing had identified the need for 'good public relations, co-operative patients, favourable home background, reasonable risk and an effective range of treatments' (Carse et al 1958). These factors remain substantially the same today, although the need to consider the desirability of home treatment for each individual (as well as just its viability), and the establishment of appropriate organisational structures, should also be highlighted.

A key contextual issue for all workers in, and planners of, mental health services is the current view of the mentally ill held within society at large, and in particular the reaction of the media to any event which appears to involve a person who has been in contact with mental health services. Philo (1998) describes a 'climate of fear' created by the media, whereby the media will focus critical attention on the providers of mental health services whenever there is a tragedy, although 'Tragedies are likely because severely mentally ill patients, whether admitted or in community care, are often dangerous to themselves and to others'.

Even bearing in mind the often one-sided and provocative nature of press coverage, there is a genuine need for providers of community-based care to consider the needs of others as well as their own clients. This is not only an acknowledgement that the wider community has a right not to be unduly distressed by disturbed behaviour, but is also based on the very practical supposition that for alternatives to admission to continue, services must have at least a modicum of good will from the general public. The White Paper *Better Services for the Mentally Ill* (HMSO 1975), made it clear that 'the demands which different groups of ill or disabled people make in total upon the community must not be greater than the community can accept'. This, of course, does not excuse either politicians and/or healthcare professionals from passively accepting misinformation or bigotry concerning the true nature of those categorised as 'mentally ill'.

Organisationally, there remains a need for medical involvement in home treatment and crisis services, both politically and in terms of providing the necessary psychiatric involvement when trying to help those with severe, acute mental health problems. Consultants remain powerful voices in healthcare organisations and it is important that there is a 'product champion' for home treatment in this forum. Home treatment services can easily be criticised and undermined if there is seen to be inadequate medical involvement and, in most areas, hospital admission remains a largely medical affair.

In order for home treatment services to be able to function successfully, resources must be adequate. Although the need for

24-hour cover may vary from area to area – with many home treatment services providing cover for shorter periods (see Orme, Chapter 2, this volume) – there is certainly a need for the staffing and financing to provide enough staff to safely cover a shift system. Furthermore the staff must be sufficiently experienced in order to cope with the demands of trying to help very disturbed individuals in a non-institutional setting. None of this is cheap. Although home treatment appears not to add overall expense, the initial funding may be problematic where there is inevitably a period before the full benefits of home treatment allow the reduction of costs in bed usage.

Fears about home treatment services

A range of concerns have been expressed concerning home treatment services:

- they may not be sustainable long-term
- they may be psychologically harmful for staff working in them
- suicide rates will increase among acute clients
- continuity of care will be adversely affected.

The results of the early research into home treatment may not be replicated in day-to-day practice: 'Studies usually recruit motivated staff, who will perform with zeal for the finite duration of the study; this may contrast with the attitudes of staff providing a routine service' (Dedman 1993). This concern has not been corroborated when financing has allowed the longer-term survival of teams (Reynolds et al 1990, Brimblecombe and O'Sullivan 1999). Teams appear to be able both to continue and to maintain clinical standards.

However, Cohen (1999) rightly points out that the history of home treatment services, and their relatively frequent dissolution, is also often related to the presence of 'key dynamic players' in the setting up and perpetuation of such services. When these individuals leave, objectives are diluted or services are amalgamated into others. Only when home treatment services become 'normalised' within the mental healthcare system and are accepted as an integral and essential part of services, as are acute admission wards, will their survival rely less on individuals (Bracken and Cohen 1999).

In terms of possible psychological damage to staff, concerns have related to the belief that the nature of providing crisis assessments and IHT will be innately stressful and potentially destructive for the staff involved: 'The rapid turnover of patients, many in great distress, inevitably puts a heavy burden on the staff of an emergency service' (Katschnig 1995). There is, as yet, no evidence to support such fears. Indeed, initial research has produced contrary results, with individual home treatment services comparing well with other mental health services in terms of stress levels (Drake and Brimblecombe 1999), job satisfaction, team identification, burnout and staff turnover (Minghella 1998).

In terms of clients' well-being, the lower levels of observation available in a community setting as compared with a hospital ward have, understandably, produced fears that home treatment may lead to increased suicide rates. However, there is also no evidence to support the concern that suicide rates may be higher in community-focused than in more hospital-focused services (Joy, Adams and Rice 1999). Working with suicidal ideation in any setting is a difficult endeavour, with occasional tragedies inevitable even when careful risk assessment takes place.

Many of the newer home treatment services provide acute, short-term interventions. Pioneering services such as those in Madison County (Stein and Test 1980) and Southwark (Marks et al 1994) provided initial intensive input to prevent admission, but also followed through the same client over an extended period. Reasonable fears have therefore been expressed as to the potential this change may have for making continuity of care difficult and providing adequate long-term follow-up.

The long-term home treatment model has obvious advantages in terms of continuity of care over an acute team model, but it also creates problems. If such services were to increase in number they would presumably need to derive from already existing community mental health teams increasing their hours, remit and staffing levels. The question has been raised as to whether simply using existing staff, in a different role with a different rationale and philosophy, is desirable. Practices and attitudes may be more easily changed when new teams are established (Minghella and Ford 1997). Extending a team's role would also involve extending its hours of working. Many existing community staff may have specifically entered such jobs to avoid doing shiftwork, for family or other reasons.

Another practical issue raised by the creation of such teams is that of the sheer size that would be required to carry out both acute and long-term follow-up functions. Arguably there is also a need for different types of staff expertise at different stages of care. Even where entirely new teams are created it seems that balancing the needs of short-term and long-term work within a single team would be extremely difficult. The answer seems to be to have separate teams with different remits, but who are closely linked managerially and in terms of day-to-day practice.

One specific advantage of specialised acute teams is that their staff will rapidly gain large amounts of experience in working with crises, and dealing with acute risk, as compared with the relatively occasional contacts with acute problems encountered by staff on a rota system (Katschnig and Konieczna 1990). An argument against this is, of course, that such specialisation will ultimately deskill staff in generic services as they routinely refer on acute and severe problems to the specialist team.

The criticism has been made that the existence of home treatment services requires that community key workers, such as social workers or CPNs, providing long-term care to their clients are made to transfer care to another team during a period of crisis (Pelosi and Jackson 2000). Any breaking of continuity of care is undesirable, yet there is no reason why this should happen. The community key worker does need to stay intimately involved in the community-based care of their client. Simply 'handing over' care to a home treatment team at crisis point should not be an option. This requires good communication between home treatment and other community teams, and ensuring that the key worker is an integral part of the home treatment care plan for the client. The Care Programme Approach provides one structure which might help in meeting this need.

A further refutation of the criticism of breaking continuity of care is, of course, that if there were no home treatment service available then the client would probably have to be admitted to hospital anyway and the links with the key worker would then be liable to be broken to a far more marked degree.

Professional resistance to home treatment

Over a long period of time doctors, clients and the general public have come to expect that serious mental disorders will be dealt with in hospitals: 'After a century and a half or more, culturally sanctioned expectations are a powerful force and are not easily modified' (Mosher 1983). 'Conventional wisdom' is therefore against major changes in delivering care, such as avoiding hospitalisation, and such thoughts are commonly found in health professionals as well as the general public. 'Clinical resistance' is still cited as a common reason preventing the development of home treatment services in some areas (Owen, Sashidharan and Edwards 2000).

Even when services are established which are able to carry out emergency assessments and provide community treatment as an alternative to admission whenever possible, it is apparent that many teams are not utilised to their full potential. Home treatment workers have repeatedly encountered professional resistance to community alternatives to admission. This has been found from the time of early services, such as that in Boston in the 1960s (Friedman et al 1964), where numerous 'loophole' admissions took place and medical staff were strongly resistant to new services, up to Devon in the 1990s where team members again believed that admissions took place 'unnecessarily' despite appropriate alternatives (Whittle and Mitchell 1997). Cohen (Chapter 8, this volume) gives a graphic account of the difficulties that can arise when home treatment teams adopt philosophies that are different, or appear to be different, from other components of mental health services.

In order to overcome such resistances various approaches are required. Friedman et al (1964) described the need to assess the 'desires and resistances' of referring professionals, moulding services to make them more acceptable with those desires and providing extensive and continual education to encourage appropriate use. However, what was ultimately successful in the case of the Boston service, described by Friedman and his colleagues, was the enforcement of a policy that all referrals for admission had to go through the home treatment service first. Subsequent experience suggests that education may not be enough and clear policies about admission and appropriate use of alternatives are essential. Home treatment services must be the gatekeepers to inpatient care in order to be effective in their role (Smyth and Hoult 2000). This is particularly important where hospital consultants are not those working directly with home treatment services.

Even when it is possible to have a policy framework supporting the principles of community-focused care and providing realistic alternatives to admission there will inevitably remain a need for negotiation with numerous other organisations. Currently the responsibility for both establishing and running community-based services is fragmented between different agencies. Each has differences in priorities, style, structure and budgets, yet they must 'request' cooperation from each other. For community care to operate effectively, these agencies must work together. There are many reasons why they fail to do so effectively, including the 'lack of positive incentives, bureaucratic barriers, perceived threats to jobs and professional standing, and the time required for interminable meetings' (Audit Commission 1986). Furthermore, conflicting ideologies can emerge between professional groups during the transition of services to those which are more community-based; these ideologies may 'complicate and indeed undermine the process' (Morgan 1992).

Home treatment services need to balance the two difficult tasks of integrating with general mental health services, whilst not losing sight of their own aims and philosophies.

The structure of home treatment/crisis services

Wide variations in the structures and practices of home treatment services exist, which cause difficulties in researching which aspects of care are most useful. However, it is likely that there is a need to tailor services to meet local needs. Inner city services, dealing predominantly with psychotic clients, clearly have different needs than those working in more rural areas.

Individuals potentially requiring urgent professional help can usefully be described in three categories (Peck and Jenkins 1992, Katschnig and Konieczna 1990):

- those in acute psychosocial crisis
- those with acute psychiatric conditions needing urgent psychiatric attention

- those with long-term, severe psychiatric problems who may experience either of the first two forms of problem.

The relative proportions of these three different client groups coming into contact with a particular emergency service will depend on many factors, including the demographics of the area the service serves (Meltzer et al 1995). Also important is the designation of the emergency service, its referral criteria, means of access, philosophy, staff skill mix and sources of funding.

Models of assessment

There exist two general models of assessment for home treatment services currently. In one the service acts as a 'crisis' assessment service itself, so the majority of urgent assessments in the area are carried out by the team who will then also provide home treatment as an alternative to admission where this is appropriate (e.g. Tufnell et al 1988, Brimblecombe and O'Sullivan 1999).

The second model is that of those services who only take referrals from psychiatrists or, occasionally, other mental health professionals (e.g. Bracken and Cohen 1999, Harrison et al 1999). Thus the initial emergency assessment is carried out, then passed to the home treatment service who will normally carry out a second assessment to verify that home treatment is as feasible as the referrer believes. There are advantages for each approach. The first ensures that assessors soon develop high levels of experience and confidence in emergency assessments. The team relies less on other professionals having a clear understanding of the role of an IHT service. Also, such services are normally more able to respond quickly and carry out assessments in a flexible manner in order to respond to clients' needs, for example seeing them in their own homes, as opposed to being seen in other common points of crisis assessment, for example Accident and Emergency departments.

A disadvantage of this model is that it may be a more expensive option. A crisis service also offering home treatment will require higher levels of staffing in order to be able to respond rapidly with a multidisciplinary assessment. Those staff will, also, need to be more experienced, and, hence, graded higher. There is a further risk, as already mentioned, that other mental health workers may be 'deskilled' by the concentration of emergency assessments being carried out by just one team. There is also the risk that, without rigorous filtering of referrals, the team could end up spending an inordinate amount of time carrying out 'inappropriate' assessments to the detriment of their home treatment function (Kwakwa 1995).

Training issues

With IHT services growing in numbers and increasingly being recognised as a key component of a comprehensive service, the mental health profession training bodies should be doing whatever they can to ensure that trainee staff gain some experience and knowledge in this area. As mentioned above, studies appear to demonstrate repeatedly that those with no experience of IHT are rarely able to adequately grasp the potential of such a service and the advantages it potentially poses for mental health clients.

In terms of the training needs of staff in home treatment services, few training programmes currently exist (see Chapter 2). Some individual areas have produced their own training programme prior to launching such a service (Minghella et al 1998), but accredited courses are rare. Working in a home treatment team is a demanding job, requiring high levels of knowledge and skills. Staff require a mixture of those attributes needed in both acute inpatient and community areas. They may carry out practical tasks, such as helping clients to attend to their own hygiene or nutritional needs, be involved in complicated negotiations with carers and other organisations, and give emotional support and psychological interventions for a wide range of difficulties. At least as important as technical skills are attitudes and the personal abilities to carry out meaningful negotiation with clients and carers. Specialist training beyond the generalities of existing community nursing or social work courses is clearly required. There now exists a store of experience and skills in this area built up, frankly, largely by trial and error over the early years of home treatment in this country. Future workers should be able to learn from their teachers' mistakes rather than their own.

A wide range of theoretical ideas are available which suggest possible areas for skills and attitude development in home treatment workers. Risk assessment training is essential in home treatment as in all areas of mental health care. Crisis intervention concepts, and ideas as to their application, may be particularly helpful for some individuals (Ratna 1978, 1982). Informal cognitive behaviourally based approaches may be useful for clients with acute psychosis (Allen and Kingdon 1998). The skills to enable staff to actively empower clients may need specific training, as this area remains underemphasised in most professionals' training. Brief therapy approaches may provide a useful tool for clarifying problems and setting goals, both for staff and clients (Drake and Brimblecombe 1999). Family interventions and specific skills in supporting carers are now recognised to be particularly important (DoH 1999b). In-depth understanding of developments in psychotropic medication and issues concerning 'compliance' (Kemp et al 1996), and related ethics, is surely essential for all professionals working with individuals with severe, acute mental health problems.

Conclusions

We are at a turning point for mental health care in the UK. Services offering IHT, linked in some form to crisis assessments, have markedly increased in number and will continue to do so in the fore-seeable future (Owen, Sashidharan and Edwards 2000; DoH 2000). Great pressure will inevitably be placed on such services to meet aims, such as reducing admission rates, but at the same time they remain vulnerable to criticism, being relatively novel forms of service.

A key dictum for all mental health services must remain that service users should be entitled to receive care in the least restrictive environment possible, and one which allows the maximum of dignity (HMSO 1999b). Without the availability of home treatment services this aim cannot be adequately realised. Philosophically there are dangers that new home treatment services may reproduce the power relations of the hospital in a community setting, especially with increasing pressure for services to be 'assertive'. This danger can be avoided, at least partially, by the principle of negotiation being at the heart of the practice of home treatment.

Inpatient services will always remain an essential part of an integrated mental health service, providing unique levels of supervision and, on occasions, containment. Hopefully, as more research becomes available, it will become clearer as to what the exact future roles of both home treatment and inpatient services will need to be.

References

Allen J, Kingdon D (1998) Using cognitive behavioural interventions for people with acute psychosis. Mental Health Practice 1(9):14–21.

Audini B, Marks I, Lawrence R, Connolly J, Watts V (1994) Home based versus outpatient/inpatient care for people with serious mental illness. Phase II of a controlled study. British Journal of Psychiatry 165:195–203.

Audit Commission (1986) Making a Reality of Community Care. London: HMSO.

Audit Commission (2000) Forget Me Not: mental health services for older people. London: Audit Commission.

Beck A, Croudace TJ, Singh S, Harrison G (1997) The Nottingham Acute Bed Study: alternatives to acute psychiatric care. British Journal of Psychiatry 170:247–252.

Bracken P, Cohen B (1999) Home treatment in Bradford. Psychiatric Bulletin 23:349–352.

Brimblecombe N (1995) The use of brief therapy as part of the nursing care plan. Nursing Times 91(35):34–35.

Brimblecombe N (2000) Suicidal ideation, home treatment and admission. Mental Health Nursing 20(1):22–26.

Brimblecombe N, O'Sullivan G (1999) Diagnosis, assessments and admissions from a community treatment team. Psychiatric Bulletin 23:72–74.

Burns T, Priebe S (1999) Mental health care failure in England. British Journal of Psychiatry 174:191–192.

Carse J, Panton NE, Watt A (1958) A District Mental Health Service. The Worthing Experiment. Lancet 4 January:39–41.

Cohen BMZ (1999) Innovatory forms of evaluation for new crisis services. Science, Discourse and Mind 1(1):12–31.

Cohen LJ, Test MA, Brown RL (1990) Suicide and schizophrenia: data from a prospective community treatment study. American Journal of Psychiatry 147(5):602–607.

Coleman M, Donnelly P, Davies A, Brace P (1998) Evaluating intensive support in community mental health care. Mental Health Nursing 18(5):8–11.

Creed FH, Black D, Anthony P, Osborn M, Thomas P, Tomenson B (1991) Day hospital for acute psychiatric illness. British Medical Journal 300:1033–1037.

Dean C, Gadd EM (1990) Home treatment for acute psychiatric illness. British Medical Journal 301:1021–1023.

Dedman P (1993) Home treatment for acute psychiatric disorder. British Medical Journal 306:1359–1360.

DoH (1998) Modernising Mental Health. Safe, sound and supportive. London: Department of Health.

DoH (1999a) Patient Care in the Community. Community psychiatric nursing: summary information for 1998–99. London: Department of Health.

DoH (1999b) National Service Framework for Mental Health. Modern standards and service models. London: Department of Health.

DoH (2000) The NHS Plan. London: Department of Health.

Drake M, Brimblecombe N (1999) Stress in mental health nursing: comparing teams. Mental Health Nursing 19(1):14–19.

Ellis J (2000) Older people bear the brunt. Mental Health Nursing 20(4):8–9.

Elwood PY (1999) Characteristics of admissions considered inappropriate by junior psychiatrists. Psychiatric Bulletin 23:34–37.

Fenton FR, Tessier L, Struening E, Smith F, Benoit C (1982) Home and Hospital Psychiatric Treatment. London: Croom Helm.

Flannigan C, Glover G, Wing J, Lewis S, Bebbington P, Feeney S (1984) Inner London collaborative audit of admission in two health districts. III: Reasons for acute admission to psychiatric wards. British Journal of Psychiatry 165:750–759.

Friedman TT, Becker A, Weiner L (1964) The psychiatric home treatment service: preliminary report of five years of clinical experience. American Journal of Psychiatry 120:782–788.

Fulop NJ, Koffman J, Carson S, Robinson A, Pashley D, Coleman K (1996) Use of acute beds: a point prevalence study in North and South Thames regions. Journal of Public Health Medicine 18(2):207–216.

Gerson S, Bassuk E (1980) Psychiatric emergencies: an overview. American Journal of Psychiatry 137(1):1–11.

Godfrey M (1996) User and carer outcomes in mental health. Outcome briefings. Nuffield Institute for Health 8:17–20.

Harrison J, Poynton A, Marshall J, Gater R, Creed F (1999) Open all hours: extending the role of the psychiatric day hospital. Psychiatric Bulletin 23:400–404.

HMSO (1975) Better Services for the Mentally Ill. Cmnd 6223. London: HMSO.

HMSO (1999a) The Health Act. London: HMSO.

HMSO (1999b) Reform of the Mental Health Act 1983. Proposals for Consultation. London: HMSO.

Hollander D, Slater MS (1994) 'Sorry, no beds': a problem for acute psychiatric admissions. Psychiatric Bulletin 18:532–534.

Hollander D, Tobiansky R, Powell R (1990) Crisis in admission beds (letter). British Medical Journal 301:664.

Holloway F (1995) Home treatment as an alternative to acute psychiatric inpatient admission: a discussion. In: Tyrer P, Creed F (eds) Community Psychiatry in Action. Analysis and prospects. Cambridge: Cambridge University Press.

Hoult J, Reynolds I, Charbonneau-Powis M, Weekes P, Briggs J (1983) Psychiatric hospital versus community treatment: the results of a randomised trial. Australian and New Zealand Journal of Psychiatry 17:160–167.

Hoult J, Rosen A, Reynolds I (1984) Community orientated treatment compared to psychiatric hospital orientated treatment. Social Science and Medicine 18(11):1005–1010.

Johnstone P, Zolese G (1999) Length of hospitalisation for people with severe mental illnesses (Cochrane Review). In: The Cochrane Library 1. Oxford: Update Software.

Joy CB, Adams CE, Rice K (1999) Crisis intervention for people with severe mental illnesses (Cochrane Review). In: The Cochrane Library 1. Oxford: Update Software.

Katschnig H (1995) The scope and limitations of emergency mental health services in the community. In: Phelan M, Strathdee G, Thornicroft G (eds) Emergency Mental Health Services in the Community. Cambridge: Cambridge University Press.

Katschnig H, Konieczna T (1990) Innovative approaches to delivery of emergency services in Europe. In: Marks IM, Scott RA, Mental Health Care Delivery: innovations, impediments and implementation. Cambridge: Cambridge University Press.

Kemp R, Hayward P, Applewhaite G, Everitt B, David A (1996) Compliance therapy in psychotic patients: randomised controlled trial. British Medical Journal 312:345–349.

Kwakwa J (1995) Alternatives to hospital-based mental health care. Nursing Times 91(23):38–39.

Langsley DG, Machotka P, Flomenhaft K (1971) Avoiding mental hospital admission: a follow-up study. American Journal of Psychiatry 127(10):127–130.

McCrone P, Chisholm D, Bould M (1999) Costing different models of mental health service provision. Mental Health Research Review 6:14–17.

McGorry PD, Chanen A, McCarthy E, Van Riel R, McKenzie D, Singh BS (1991) Posttraumatic stress disorder following recent-onset psychosis. An unrecognized postpsychotic syndrome. Journal of Nervous and Mental Disease 179(5):253–258.

Marks IM, Connolly J, Muijen M, Audini B, McNamee G, Lawrence RE (1994) Home-based versus hospital-based care for people with serious mental illness. British Journal of Psychiatry 165:179–194.

Meltzer H, Gil B, Petticrew M, Hinds K (1995) The Prevalence of Psychiatric Morbidity among Adults Living in Private Households. London: HMSO.

Minghella E (1998) Home-based emergency treatment. Mental Health Practice 2(1):10–14.

Minghella E, Ford R (1997) All for one and one for all? Health Service Journal 13 March:30–31.

Minghella E, Ford R, Freeman T, Hoult J, McGlynn P, O'Halloran P (1998) Open All Hours. 24-hour response for people with mental health emergencies. London: Sainsbury Centre for Mental Health.

Moore C, Wolf J (1999) Open and shut case. Health Service Journal 24 June:20–22.

Morgan G (1992) Suicide prevention. Hazards on the fast lane to community care. British Journal of Psychiatry 160:149–153.

Mosher LR (1983) Alternatives to psychiatric hospitalization. Why has research failed to be translated into practice? New England Journal of Medicine 309(25):1579–1580.

Mountain G (1998) The delivery of community mental health services to older people. Mental Health Review 3(1):7–15.

Muijen M, Cooney M, Strathdee G, Bell R, Hudson A (1994) Community psychiatric nurse teams: intensive support versus generic care. British Journal of Psychiatry 165:211–217.

Owen AJ, Sashidharan SP, Edwards LJ (2000) Availability and acceptability of home treatment for acute psychiatric disorders. Psychiatric Bulletin 24:169–171.

Pasamanick B, Scarpitti FR, Dinitz S (1967) Schizophrenics in the Community: an experimental study in the prevention of hospitalization. New York: Appleton-Century-Crofts.

Peck E, Jenkins J (1992) The development of acute psychiatric crisis services in England: Opportunities, problems and trends. Journal of Mental Health 1:193–200.

Pelosi A, Jackson GA (2000) Home treatment – enigmas and failures. British Medical Journal 320:308–309.

Philo G (1998) The media and mental health promotion. Mental Health Review 3(2):21–25.

Ratna L (1978) The Practice of Psychiatric Crisis Intervention. St Albans: Napsbury Hospital League of Friends.

Ratna L (1982) Crisis intervention in psychogeriatrics: a two-year follow-up study. British Journal of Psychiatry 141:296–301.

Reynolds I, Jones JE, Berry DW, Hoult JE (1990) A crisis team for the mentally ill: the effect on patients, relatives and admissions. Medical Journal of Australia 152:646–652.

Richardson K (1989) Locally based community care. A personal view. Psychiatric Bulletin 13:287–290.

Sainsbury Centre for Mental Health (1998) Acute Problems. A survey of the quality of life in acute psychiatric wards. London: Sainsbury Centre for Mental Health.

Sashidharan SP (1999) Alternatives to institutional psychiatry. In: Bhugra D, Bal V (eds) Ethnicity: an agenda for mental health. London: Gaskell.

Sayce L, Craig TKJ, Boardman AP (1991) The development of community mental health centres in the UK. Social Psychiatry and Psychiatric Epidemiology 26:14–20.

Smyth M, Bracken P (1994) Senior registrar training in home treatment. Psychiatric Bulletin 18:408–409.

Smyth MG, Hoult J (2000) The home treatment enigma. British Medical Journal 320:305–307.

Spencer G, Jolley D (1999) Planning services for the elderly. Advances in Psychiatric Treatment 5:202–212.

Stein L, Test MA (1980) Alternative to mental hospital treatment: I. Conceptual model, treatment program, and clinical expectation. Archives of General Psychiatry 37:392–397.

Stephens H, Huws R (1997) Making the right link. Health Service Journal. 2 October: 32–33.

Taylor PJ, Gunn J (1999) Homicides by people with mental illness: myth and reality. British Journal of Psychiatry 174:9–14.

Thompson R (1999) Home care of the elderly with mental health needs. Nursing Times 95(10):48–49.

Trieman N, Leff J, Glover G (1999) Outcome of long stay psychiatric patients resettled in the community: prospective cohort study. British Medical Journal 319:13–16.

Tufnell G, Bouras N, Watson JP, Brough DI (1988) Home assessment and treatment in a community psychiatric service. Acta Psychiatrica Scandinavica 72:20–28.

Whittle P, Mitchell S (1997) Community alternatives project: An evaluation of a community-based acute psychiatric team providing alternatives to admission. Journal of Mental Health 6(4):417–427.

Williams DDR, Ellis ME, Hardwick F (1997) Intensive home nursing. An innovation in old age psychiatry. Psychiatric Bulletin 21:23–25.

Wood H (1994) What do service users want from mental health services? Report to the Audit Commission for Finding a Place: a Review of Mental Health Services for Adults. London: HMSO.

Wykes T, Leese M, Taylor R et al (1998) Effects of community services on disability and symptoms. PRiSM Psychosis Study 4. British Journal of Psychiatry 173:385–390.

Index